Mobile Communication in Asia: Local Insights, Global Implications

Series editor
Sun Sun Lim, Department of Communications and New Media,
National University of Singapore, Singapore

More information about this series at http://www.springer.com/series/13350

Sun Sun Lim
Editor

Mobile Communication and the Family

Asian Experiences in Technology Domestication

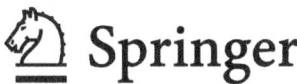 Springer

Editor
Sun Sun Lim
Department of Communications and New Media
National University of Singapore
Singapore

ISSN 2468-2403 ISSN 2468-2411 (electronic)
Mobile Communication in Asia: Local Insights, Global Implications
ISBN 978-94-017-7439-0 ISBN 978-94-017-7441-3 (eBook)
DOI 10.1007/978-94-017-7441-3

Library of Congress Control Number: 2015958725

Springer Dordrecht Heidelberg New York London
© Springer Science+Business Media Dordrecht 2016
This work is subject to copyright. All rights are reserved by the Publisher, whether the whole or part of the material is concerned, specifically the rights of translation, reprinting, reuse of illustrations, recitation, broadcasting, reproduction on microfilms or in any other physical way, and transmission or information storage and retrieval, electronic adaptation, computer software, or by similar or dissimilar methodology now known or hereafter developed.
The use of general descriptive names, registered names, trademarks, service marks, etc. in this publication does not imply, even in the absence of a specific statement, that such names are exempt from the relevant protective laws and regulations and therefore free for general use.
The publisher, the authors and the editors are safe to assume that the advice and information in this book are believed to be true and accurate at the date of publication. Neither the publisher nor the authors or the editors give a warranty, express or implied, with respect to the material contained herein or for any errors or omissions that may have been made.

Printed on acid-free paper

Springer Science+Business Media B.V. Dordrecht is part of Springer Science+Business Media (www.springer.com)

To my family, with love and affection

Acknowledgements

I am tremendously grateful to the many families and individuals whose experiences are captured in this volume. Their candid views, deep reflections and personal encounters with technology have brought us closer to understanding how mobile communication is insinuating its way into our daily lives. As well, these families' rich experiences would remain unknown to academia without the scholarship of this volume's contributors. I have benefited considerably from their insights and analyses and look forward to learning from their future research endeavours.

I am also indebted to the community of scholars whose research on technology adoption in the domestic realm has informed and inspired my work in this area. Special thanks are owed to the father of technology domestication himself, the late Roger Silverstone. I am much obliged to the editorial team at Springer, Jayanthie Krishnan and Vishal Daryanomel, for their prompt and cheerful assistance throughout the entire process from proposal to publication. I owe a debt of gratitude to my stupendous research assistants, Kakit Cheong, Loh Sze Ming and Becky Pham, whose energy and industry never fail to impress me.

Most of all, I thank my wonderful husband Jin and my two lovely children Kai Ryn and Kai Wyn, whose questions about technology always trigger my 'aha' moments!

Contents

1   Asymmetries in Asian Families' Domestication
    of Mobile Communication 1
    Sun Sun Lim

Part I Values

2   Desiring Mobiles, Desiring Education: Mobile Phones
    and Families in a Rural Chinese Town 13
    Tom McDonald

3   Balancing Religion, Technology and Parenthood: Indonesian
    Muslim Mothers' Supervision of Children's Internet Use 33
    Rahayu and Sun Sun Lim

4   Helping the Helpers: Understanding Family Storytelling
    by Domestic Helpers in Singapore 51
    Kakit Cheong and Alex Mitchell

Part II Intimacies

5   Mobile Technology and "Doing Family" in a Global
    World: Indian Migrants in Cambodia 73
    Ravinder Kaur and Ishita Shruti

6   The Cultural Appropriation of Smartphones in Korean
    Transnational Families 93
    Kyong Yoon

7   Empowering Interactions, Sustaining Ties: Vietnamese
    Migrant Students' Communication with Left-Behind
    Families and Friends 109
    Becky Pham and Sun Sun Lim

Part III Strategies

8   Restricting, Distracting, and Reasoning: Parental Mediation of Young Children's Use of Mobile Communication Technology in Indonesia... 129
Laras Sekarasih

9   Paradoxes in the Mobile Parenting Experiences of Filipino Mothers in Diaspora.. 147
Ma. Rosel S. San Pascual

10 The Value of the Life Course Perspective in the Design of Mobile Technologies for Older Adults 165
Pin Sym Foong

Index.. 183

About the Authors

Kakit Cheong is an MA candidate in the Department of Communications and New Media, National University of Singapore. His current research explores how information and communication technologies can be designed to support family storytelling for migrant workers. His recent work includes 'Kwento: using a participatory approach to designing a family storytelling application for domestic helpers' (with Alex Mitchell, for the International Conference on Human-Computer Interaction, 2015).

Pin Sym Foong has an MSc in human-computer interaction design and is currently pursuing her PhD at the School of Integrative Sciences and Engineering in the National University of Singapore. Her current project focuses on supporting the visitor-nursing home resident relationship with technologies that enable social interaction and cognitive stimulation. Previously, she was a lecturer in human-computer interaction, mobile interaction and user experience design, where she guided her students towards winning several international HCI design competitions. Her work with older adults is supported by her experience as an interface developer for multimedia services and as a mentor to new media start-ups.

Ravinder Kaur is professor of sociology and social anthropology in the Department of Humanities and Social Sciences, Indian Institute of Technology Delhi, New Delhi, India. She earlier taught at Delhi University and New York University. Her areas of interest are kinship, family, marriage, gender, migration and social change. Besides publishing numerous articles on these topics, she has recently coedited the book *Marrying in South Asia: Shifting Concepts, Changing Practices in a Globalising World* (with Rajni Palriwala), published in 2014 by Orient Blackswan. She has two other books under preparation: *Too Many Men, Too Few Women: Social Consequences of the Gender Imbalance in India and China* and *Strangers as Spouses: Skewed Sex Ratios and Marriage Migration in India*.

Sun Sun Lim (PhD, London School of Economics) is associate professor at the Department of Communications and New Media and assistant dean for research at the Faculty of Arts and Social Sciences, National University of Singapore. She studies the social implications of technology domestication by young people and families, charting the ethnographies of their internet and mobile phone use and publishing more than 50 monographs, journal articles and book chapters. Her recent research has focused attention on understudied and marginalised populations including juvenile delinquents, youths-at-risk and migrant workers. She serves on the editorial boards of the *Journal of Computer Mediated Communication*; *Journal of Children and Media*; *Communication, Culture & Critique*; and *Mobile Media & Communication*.

Tom McDonald is an assistant professor in the Department of Sociology at the University of Hong Kong. Prior to this he was a research associate in the Department of Anthropology, University College London, where he conducted 15 months of ethnographic fieldwork in rural China, studying the impact of social media use amongst local people as part of the Global Social Media Impact Study. Tom received his PhD in anthropology from University College London in 2013, which investigated the migration of hospitality practices in a south-western Chinese town, charting its movement from the domestic sphere to new commercial venues outside the home.

Alex Mitchell is an assistant professor in the Department of Communications and New Media at the National University of Singapore. His current research investigates various aspects of computer-based art and entertainment, focusing in particular on interactive stories in digital and nondigital interactive storytelling systems. His recent publications include 'Telling stories on the go: lessons from a mobile thematic storytelling system' (with Teong Leong Chuah, in *Lecture Notes in Computer Science*, 2013, volume 8230/2013, *Interactive Storytelling*, 2013), 'Rereading as echo: a close (re)reading of Emily Short's *A Family Supper*' (in *ISSUE: Art Journal*, 2, 2013) and 'Defamiliarization and poetic interaction in *Kentucky Route Zero*' (in *Well Played Journal*, 3 (2), ETC Press, 2014). He was the general chair for the International Conference on Interactive Digital Storytelling (ICIDS), 2014, and is a member of the ICIDS steering committee.

Becky Pham is an MA candidate at the Department of Communications and New Media, National University of Singapore. She has a keen research interest in studying how young people appropriate new media and technology and how their technology engagement shapes their world view. Her other research interests include media and migration, media representations, human-computer interactions and out-of-home television.

Rahayu is a lecturer in the Department of Communication Studies, Faculty of Social and Political Sciences, Universitas Gadjah Mada, Indonesia. She is currently a full-time PhD student in the Department of Public Policy and Management in the same university. She teaches several subjects, namely, media management, community relations, public opinion and quantitative research methods. She is interested in the study of media industry, media and communication policy, media performance, local media, media users and media literacy. Her research and articles have been published in newspapers, magazines, monographs, proceedings, academic journals and several edited volumes.

Ma. Rosel S. San Pascual is a full-time faculty member of the Department of Communication Research of the College of Mass Communication, University of the Philippines. She has a graduate degree in communications and new media from the National University of Singapore. Her recent research focuses on transnational migration, family communication and new media. She teaches courses on quantitative research at both undergraduate and graduate levels.

Laras Sekarasih (PhD, University of Massachusetts Amherst, 2015) is a postdoctoral associate at the University of Massachusetts Amherst Institute for Social Science Research. Her research interests are media, children, and the family, media literacy and media and consumers. Her dissertation examined the relationship between parents' television viewing and the cultivation of materialism amongst families with young adult offspring. Her work has appeared in the *Journal of Children and Media* and the *Journal of Media Literacy Education*. A recent work on the use of media literacy education to promote critical thinking about cyberbullying amongst 6th graders in Frechette, J., & Williams, R. (Eds). *Media Education for a Digital Generation*. New York: Routledge.

Ishita Shruti is visiting faculty in the Department of Public Health, State University of Bangladesh, Dhaka. She holds a PhD from the Department of Humanities and Social Sciences, Indian Institute of Technology Delhi. Her areas of interest are migration and gender. She has been closely involved with many academic and social research initiatives in the areas of gender, migration and urban governance. She has presented papers in various national and international conferences in Asia and Europe. She has extensive experience working with national and international development organisations in India and Cambodia. Her professional strengths lie in research, advocacy and networking.

Kyong Yoon is an assistant professor in cultural studies at the University of British Columbia Okanagan, Canada. His research interests are transnational mobility, digital mobile communication and transnational media audience. His recent research project concerns Korean immigrants' use of new media in Canada. He also studies the cultural implications of cross-cultural media flows with reference to Korean pop culture in North America. He is an editorial board member of *Asiascape: Digital Asia*.

Chapter 1
Asymmetries in Asian Families' Domestication of Mobile Communication

Sun Sun Lim

Abstract As powerful, portable media devices such as smartphones and tablets diffuse across the region at an unparalleled rate, families in Asia are coming to terms with the many asymmetries that these gadgets herald. Because mobile communication devices are deeply personal, but are also vested with a remarkable combination of instrumentality and emotionality, their entry into a household will inevitably provoke alternating reactions of anticipation and dread, efficacy and inadequacy, liberation and enslavement, and joy and drudgery. Within every home, these emotional dualities will pervade each family member's experience of domesticating mobile devices, making asymmetries relating to power, expectations, practice, access, competencies, and values increasingly palpable. Families must therefore negotiate such asymmetries as they manage the growing presence of mobile communication devices and their expanding repertoire of locative and social media functions.

Keywords Families • Mobile communication • Negotiation • Strategies • Values

A low-waged Indian migrant worker in Cambodia diligently saves up to buy his wife back home a mobile phone, thus raising her status among her in-laws. A mother in Vietnam demands that her daughter, a university student in Singapore, be constantly contactable by phone. A toddler in Indonesia knows that if she wants to play games on a mobile device, she will have greater luck approaching her father than her mother.

What do these families from diverse parts of Asia, avidly incorporating mobile communication into their daily lives, have in common? In a word, asymmetries. As powerful, portable media devices such as smartphones and tablets diffuse across the region at an unparalleled rate, families in Asia are coming to terms with the many asymmetries that these gadgets herald. The simple matter of who owns or pays for

S.S. Lim (✉)
Department of Communications and New Media,
National University of Singapore, Singapore
e-mail: sunlim@nus.edu.sg

a mobile device can introduce power asymmetries in a family, enabling one member to impose conditions on another. Expectation asymmetries have also emerged with regard to one's contactability, with some parents demanding that their children respond to every call or message and some children perceiving such intrusions as surveillance. Practice asymmetries also result when parents (and extended family) inconsistently apply rules surrounding children's use of mobile devices.

Many more asymmetries abound, such as those pertaining to access, competencies and values. Access asymmetries are characteristic of transnational families, where the family member residing abroad often enjoys higher standards of connectivity than those back home, and must resourcefully bridge the gap to ensure seamless communication. Even when access divides can be narrowed, competency asymmetries persist wherein some family members simply lack the technical skills to benefit from the affordances of more advanced channels of information and communication. Value asymmetries are also evident when family members cannot agree on whether mobile communication devices are the gateway to knowledge and academic achievement or the path to deleterious distraction.

My focus on asymmetries is a deliberate one. Because mobile communication devices are deeply personal, but are also vested with a remarkable combination of instrumentality and emotionality, their entry into a household will inevitably provoke alternating reactions of anticipation and dread, efficacy and inadequacy, liberation and enslavement and joy and drudgery. Within every home, these emotional dualities will pervade, in varying degrees, each family member's experience of domesticating mobile devices, making the asymmetries even more palpable. Families in Asia are constantly negotiating such asymmetries, developing strategies to manage the growing presence of mobile communication devices and their expanding repertoire of locative and social media functions. No aspect of family life is untouched by mobile communication as households employ its myriad affordances for communication, information, entertainment, the nurturance of familial bonds and the organisation of everyday routines.

The significant impact of mobile communication in Asia thus justifies a book that focuses on this disruptive technology, but from the perspective of the family. However, just as mobile communication constantly evolves, families in Asia are also experiencing significant changes in light of unprecedented economic growth, globalisation, urbanisation and demographic shifts (Hennon and Wilson 2008). Asia is therefore at the crossroads of technological transformation and social change, and this book aims to capture the interactions of these two contemporaneous trends. This collection showcases research on Asian families across a spectrum of socioeconomic profiles, from both rural and urban areas, offering perspectives on children, adolescents, adults and the elderly. As well, the different chapters feature a range of family types including nuclear, multigenerational, transnational and multilocal, spanning the continuum from the media-rich to the media have-less. These families' varied yet convergent experiences illuminate how mobile communication is influencing family interactions and shaping the bonds on which familial relationships are built.

Technology Domestication in the Mobile Age

Undeniably, mobile communication devices have inveigled their way into the domestic space, to the point of being "taken for granted" (Ling 2012). Yet the impact that these devices have on families can hardly be taken for granted, much less unquestioningly accepted. As Clark (2014) observed, mobile media "mediate, symbolise, and disrupt or reinforce the social relations of the family" (p. 329). In this regard, technology domestication offers a valuable conceptual apparatus for understanding the superimposition of technological structures over the complexities of family dynamics.

Now into its fourth decade, the concept of technology domestication can truly come into its own, in an era where mobile communication devices have embedded computing power and internet connectivity into more households than ever before. As both an analytical framework and a methodological approach, technology domestication was a significant departure from earlier "rational, linear, monocausal and technologically determined" (Berker et al. 2006, p. 1) frames of studying technology adoption. Instead, the concept exhorts researchers to look beyond the transactional and procedural dimensions of technology adoption and to focus on the intangible aspects of what is fundamentally an individualised, amorphous and haphazard process. In so doing, researchers can distil the meanings that users inscribe in and ascribe to technologies by capturing their narratives and interpretations.

Much has been written about the four processes that occur when a technology is introduced into a household: *appropriation*, *objectification*, *incorporation* and *conversion* (Silverstone et al. 1992), but a brief review here would be appropriate. Broadly, the concept argues that objectification and incorporation take place within the internal realm of the household, while appropriation and conversion extend the boundaries of the household into the outside world. In appropriation, individuals or households take possession of objects and assign them meanings. Objectification is also likely to occur, where these objects are subsequently used or displayed in the home, thus embodying the values of their owners and users. Incorporation is the process by which objects are integrated into the quotidian rhythms of the household, performing both affective and mechanical functions. Conversion in turn connects the household's moral economy with the public sphere, and information and communication technologies (ICTs) exist as both objects and facilitators of conversion (and conversation).

All these processes take place against the backdrop of the moral economy of the household. Silverstone et al. referred to it as "an economy of meanings and a meaningful economy" (1992, p. 18) wherein the household is an economic unit in its own right, ordering its economic and social activities according to a set of shared values and beliefs. Therefore, through the production and consumption activities of family members, the household becomes a part of the public economy. These economic activities within the household and the larger public economy are in turn influenced by the morals undergirding the family.

As a concept, technology domestication has had considerable reach, having been applied to the study of different family contexts in Europe and North America including nuclear families (e.g. Hirsch 1992) and single-parent households (e.g. Haddon and Silverstone 1995), shedding light on parent–child relationships (e.g. Pasquier 2001) and gender roles (e.g. Frissen 1997) vis-à-vis ICTs. Previous research has also targeted specific age groups, including children (e.g. Livingstone 2002), young adults (e.g. Hartmann 2005) and the elderly (e.g. Haddon and Silverstone 1996). With regard to the technological devices/services studied, some studies took an encompassing approach by including all technologies within the home, while others focused on a single technological device such as the computer (e.g. Aune 1996), or the internet (e.g. Bakardjieva 2005). When I first began my research on technology domestication by Chinese and Korean households (Lim 2006, 2008), the concept had not been widely applied to Asian contexts. Previous research on technology appropriation in the home had been conducted, although not necessarily informed by the domestication framework, such as in China (notably, Lull 1991), Japan (e.g. Kanayama 2003), Korea (e.g. Yoon 2003) and Singapore (e.g. Lim and Tan 2004).

Despite the broad range of its application, several aspects of technology domestication have been found wanting. Early criticisms that domestication tended to study only conventional families (parents with children in close propinquity) have since been addressed with research on a mutiplicity of family types and constitutions, including in this volume. Further suggestions for refinement include a sharpened focus on the "emotional work" that drives the moral economy of the family (Clark 2014). A more persistent issue with domestication research relates to the "double articulation" of media as "specific technologies: they are both objects and conveyer of messages" (Hartmann 2006, p. 85). The challenge then is to comprehensively examine media content in tandem with the media context and to effectively analyse their mutual interactions. Existing research tends to privilege one dimension over the other, with few being able to successfully study both in equal measure. To be sure, methodological constraints and ethical concerns prevent more sustained and invasive fieldwork that can facilitate greater insight into the untidy complexities of the domestic realm. The studies featured in this volume utilise a range of methods including interviews, ethnography, observation, diaries, cultural probes and media deprivation. By critically assessing each of these methods and the data they yield for their respective settings, we can seek to develop a methodological matrix that outlines the relative strengths and weaknesses of each research approach for studying the adoption of mobile communication, so that both content and context can be well captured. Such efforts will help to resolve this perennial concern of technology domestication research.

Values/Intimacies/Strategies

While not all of the chapters in this volume apply the concept of technology domestication, they have embraced its spirit of exploring the meaning that mobile communication holds for families, beyond a mere account of its practical benefits and costs. The chapters are organised according to three themes: values, intimacies and strategies, although there are many instances where all three themes intersect in interesting ways.

The three chapters in the first section centre around the *values* that form the core of families' moral economies. Tom McDonald (Chap. 2) studied the use of mobile phones in a rural Chinese town, examining the relationship between mobile communication technologies and education. His ethnographic data shows that for these rural families, education is the springboard for upward mobility and is consequently their foremost priority. His findings demonstrate how the mobile phone is the veritable lens through which societal valorisation of educational achievement is reflected and indeed refracted, illuminating how these everyday devices are not merely with vested technological capacity, but laden with cultural values. Parents in rural environments view mobile phones, with their countless diversions, as inimical to their children's academic pursuits and therefore to be restricted. But the young people find creative ways to circumvent such controls and actively use mobile phones, recognising that these devices are indispensable for social networking, a key aspect of education that they find their parents woefully ignorant of.

In contrast, the Muslim mothers in suburban Indonesia, studied by Rahayu and Sun Sun Lim (Chap. 3), are well aware of the growing importance of technology and want their children to be IT literate. However, they also fear that negative online content may lead to moral degradation, spiritual corruption and self-destruction in their children. Hence, they seek to balance their practical outlook with their religious ideals by allowing their children internet access while imposing mediation heavily informed by their faith. In Muslim families, mothers are tasked with socialising children on Islamic beliefs and values, and these women use their religious principles as a bulwark against the perceived harms of online content. Their experience is indeed one of taming "wild technologies", the metaphor that lends the concept of technology domestication its name.

However, with domestication comes compliance, and previously alien technologies can be coaxed into the service of the family, to aid in the nurturance of familial ties and the inculcation of cherished values. Kakit Cheong and Alex Mitchell (Chap. 4) studied Filipino domestic helpers working in Singapore, asking them what stories they told their family members back home and how they deployed mobile technologies in this process. Family storytelling is known to help families maintain close bonds, shape shared identities and even overcome adversity. Although these domestic helpers work in restrictive conditions, they nevertheless marshal their limited mobile phone access to tell family members stories that help to make sense of their physical separation and to instil family values and Christian doctrine in their left-behind children.

For transnational families in particular, whether their interaction relates to the lofty inculcation of values or to mundane daily updates, mobile communication is crucial for forging *intimacies* and nourishing relationships. The three chapters in the second section focus on such intimacies. Ravinder Kaur and Ishita Shruti (Chap. 5) sought to understand how rural and urban transnational families are "doing family" with mobile communication. They compared two groups of Indian migrants working in Cambodia – rural and less educated single male migrants working as itinerant street vendors and highly educated professionals working in white collar jobs, some of whose family members are scattered around the globe. The authors found that because education, income levels and the cost of technologies shape these migrants' access to technologies, professionals can avail of more advanced technologies while the rural migrants make do with more basic facilities. Across the two groups, however, more regular communication enables them to nurture deep affective bonds that help them to approximate, if not experience, the "family feeling". For the rural migrants in particular, mobile communication is the conduit for renewing ties with the culture of their homeland and for expressing care through sending remittances to the family. For the professionals, multiple forms of mobile communication are exploited so that their multilocal families can experience virtual togetherness despite being geographically dispersed.

Indeed, the emotional geographies of transnational families can often be as complex as their physical geographies. Kyong Yoon (Chap. 6) explored the communication practices of South Korean families whose young adult children reside in Canada, while their parents remained mostly in Korea. For these young people who had emigrated in their teen years, being apart from their parents is a reality they have become accustomed to over many years. Their default mode of interaction with their parents is via online channels and some even prefer mediated to face-to-face interaction. They utilise a range of smartphone-enabled services including KakaoTalk (messaging app), KakaoStory (for selfies and status updates), Facebook, and video calls via Skype to enhance the sense of copresence and to foster a sense of belonging in the family. There is a fondness for 'visual technologies' such as video calls and photographs that make it possible to 'see' one another, as well as the use of humorous and cute emoticons to mediate tensions in online communication. Even so, some respondents decry the misunderstandings that occasionally arise from mediated interaction. Besides communication, parents also leverage smartphone functions for mobile parenting, with mothers in particular using KakaoTalk to keep a watchful eye over their children's daily activities even across the miles.

Similarly, Vietnamese parents whose children are pursuing university studies in Singapore also exercise parental oversight via mobile communication and social media. Becky Pham and Sun Sun Lim (Chap. 7) investigated these Vietnamese migrant students' communication with their left-behind families and found that such remote supervision, while born out of parental care and concern, is perceived by the children as unwelcome surveillance. However, these students grudgingly accept rather than actively resist such interference, recognising that their parents' constant mediated presence helps cushion them from the challenges of adapting to their host country. They experienced this acutely when the study's media deprivation condition required that they cease communicating with their left-behind families for one week. Most of the students were negatively affected by this loss of contact, feeling sad and distressed at the absence of their parents' emotional support and anxious from not knowing about the well-being of their loved ones. Notably, however, this deprivation experience also highlighted to some students the need to lean less on their parents and to develop emotional independence.

Ultimately therefore, all families that appropriate mobile communication are aware of their impact on household dynamics and consciously or instinctively develop *strategies* to manage the same, the theme uniting the remaining three chapters. Laras Sekarasih (Chap. 8) probed parents of preschoolers in Indonesia to understand how they mediated their children's smartphone and tablet use. While these parents appreciate the educational, entertainment and "child-minding" benefits of these devices, they feel that health risks, such as eyestrain and physical inactivity, and exposure to violent or sexually explicit content far outweigh the gains. Most parents interviewed thus practise restrictive mediation on duration and content, actively mediate by reasoning with the children or steer them towards alternative diversions. Effective mediation is, however, an ongoing challenge as both parents may not be equally strict with the children, or other caregivers in the home are simply too permissive. In multigenerational settings, older family members such as grandparents tend to be quick to indulge the children's requests for mobile device access, thereby driving a wedge between parents and grandparents.

Navigating between the boon and bane of mobile communication is therefore a salient thread coursing through the experiences of the many families featured in this volume. Rosel San Pascual (Chap. 9) deals squarely with this issue by focusing on the paradoxes surrounding the mobile communication of Filipino migrant mothers of teenaged children who were working in Singapore. She identifies three main paradoxes: independence/dependence, competence/incompetence and empowerment/enslavement, uncovering the equivocation with which these women use mobile communication for remote parenting. While they treasure the independence that mobile communication grants them, enabling them to work overseas while remaining connected to family, they also resent the degree to which they are dependent on it. Indeed, they feel as much empowered by and enslaved to these digital connections. Fundamentally, their negative feelings are rooted in the doubts clouding over their own parenting. While gratified that they can parent from a distance, they are also overwhelmed by societal expectations that only the mother who is by her children's side is the proverbial good mother (see also Soriano et al. 2015 on Philippine media representations that reinforce such norms). Despite such misgivings, these women convince themselves that through the strategic use of mobile communication, they can parent effectively and reach the best compromise for themselves and their children.

At every stage of the family's development, therefore, from when the children are very young, through to their adolescence and emerging adulthood, families seek to manage and exploit mobile communication in the interest of positive household dynamics. The book thus concludes with an important prescription on how mobile technologies can be harnessed for the care of older adults. Pin Sym Foong (Chap. 10) makes a compelling case for taking a life course perspective in human–computer interaction design for the elderly, proposing a Gerotech Clock that depicts how the needs of older users vis-à-vis mobile technology evolve over time. She also urges designers to be conscious of the distinction between age, life stage and cohort effects, because each factor would influence elderly users' technological competencies and adoption tendencies. She argues that when the elderly are relatively free from physical impairment, mobile technology can be crafted to enhance their independence. But once the elderly become reliant on caregivers from within and outside of the family, technology design must take into account the needs and constraints of all parties, while being sensitive to their relationship dynamics. She ends by challenging designers to cater to the complex needs of ageing societies in our increasingly mobile landscape.

About This Book Series

Putting this book together has been gratifying in many ways. I had long recognised the relative paucity of published research on mobile communication in Asia, despite the technology's growing importance in the region (Lim and Goggin 2014). At the same time, I was also aware of the vast number of researchers in the region whose innovative work had yet to be published in the customary anglophone outlets, thereby circumscribing their contributions to the broader academic mission – investigating the social impact of technology. In developing this book series, I aim to showcase the work of emerging scholars for the wider international audience, thereby introducing fresh perspectives to the global conversation on the transformative effect of mobile communication. Hence, the series is entitled *Mobile Communication in Asia: Local Insights, Global Implications*. I am heartened that Springer appreciates the merits of this endeavour and has thrown its support behind the series, as have many colleagues who have committed to editing future volumes. In editing this first volume in the series, I have had the privilege of mentoring and learning from emerging scholars whose ground insights and diverse perspectives will help to advance our understanding of Asia's increasingly complex sociotechnical morphology. Their valuable contributions also signal that research on mobile communication in Asia is set to make a long-term impact, both within the region and beyond.

References

Aune, M. (1996). The computer in everyday life: Patterns of domestication of a new technology. In M. Lie & K. Sorensen (Eds.), *Making technology our own? Domesticating technology into everyday life* (pp. 91–120). Oslo: Scandinavian University Press.

Bakardjieva, M. (2005). *Internet society: The internet in everyday life*. London: Sage.

Berker, T., Hartmann, M., Punie, Y., & Ward, K. (2006). Introduction. In T. Berker, M. Hartmann, Y. Punie & K. J. Ward (Eds.), *Domestication of media and technology* (pp. 1–17). Maidenhead: Open University Press.

Clark, L. S. (2014). Mobile media in the emotional and moral economies of the household. In G. Goggin & L. Hjorth (Eds.), *Routledge companion to mobile media* (pp. 320–332). London: Routledge.

Frissen, V. (1997). *Gender, ICTs and everyday life: Mutual shaping processes*. Brussels: European Commission.

Haddon, L., & Silverstone, R. (1995). *Lone parents and their information and communication technologies*. SPRU/CICT report series no. 12. Falmer, Sussex: University of Sussex.

Haddon, L., & Silverstone, R. (1996). *Information and communication technologies and the young elderly*. SPRU/CICT report series no. 13. Falmer, Sussex: University of Sussex.

Hartmann, M. (2005). The discourse of the perfect future – Young people and new technologies. In R. Silverstone (Ed.), *Media, technology and everyday life* (pp. 141–158). Aldershot: Ashgate.

Hartmann, M. (2006). The triple articulation of ICTs. Media as technological objects, symbolic environments and individual texts. In T. Berker, M. Hartmann, Y. Punie & K. J. Ward (Eds.), *Domestication of media and technology* (pp. 80–102). Maidenhead: Open University Press.

Hennon, C. B., & Wilson, S. M. (2008). Families in global context: Understanding diversity through comparative analysis. In C. B. Hennon & S. M. Wilson (Eds.), *Families in a global context* (pp. 1–14). New York: Routledge.

Hirsch, E. (1992). The long term and the short term of domestic consumption. In R. Silverstone & E. Hirsch (Eds.), *Consuming technologies* (pp. 208–226). London: Routledge.

Kanayama, T. (2003). Ethnographic research on the experience of Japanese elderly people online. *New Media and Society, 5*(2), 267–288.

Lim, S. S. (2006). From cultural to information revolution: ICT domestication by middle-class families in urban China. In M. Hartmann, T. Berker, Y. Punie & K. Ward (Eds.), *Domestication of media and technology* (pp. 185–204). Maidenhead: Open University Press.

Lim, S. S. (2008) Technology domestication in the Asian homestead: Comparing the experiences of middle class families in China and South Korea. *East Asian Science, Technology and Society, 2*(2), 1875–2160.

Lim, S. S., & Goggin, G. (2014). Mobile communication in Asia: Issues and imperatives. *Journal of Computer Mediated Communication, 19*(3), 663–666.

Lim, S. S., & Tan, Y. L. (2004) Parental control of new Media usage – The challenges of Infocomm illiteracy. *Australian Journal of Communication, 31*(1), 57–74.

Ling, R. (2012). *Taken for grantedness: The embedding of mobile communication into society*. Cambridge, MA: MIT Press.

Livingstone, S. (2002). *Young people and new media*. London: Sage.

Lull, J. (1991). *China turned on: Television, reform and resistance*. London: Routledge.

Pasquier, D. (2001). Media at home: Domestic interactions and regulation. In S. Livingstone & M. Bovill (Eds.), *Children and their changing environment: A european comparative study* (pp. 161–179). Mahwah: Lawrence Erlbaum Associates.

Silverstone, R., Hirsch, E., & Morley, D. (1992). Information and communication technologies and the moral economy of the household. In R. Silverstone & E. Hirsch (Eds.), *Consuming technologies* (pp. 15–31). London: Routledge.

Soriano, C., Lim, S. S., & Rivera, M. (2015). The Virgin Mary with a mobile phone – Representations of mothering and mobile consumption in Philippine television advertisements. *Communication, Culture & Critique, 8*(11), 1–19.

Yoon, K. (2003). Retraditionalising the mobile: Young people's sociality and mobile phone use in Seoul, South Korea. *European Journal of Cultural Studies, 6*(3), 327–343.

Part I
Values

Chapter 2
Desiring Mobiles, Desiring Education: Mobile Phones and Families in a Rural Chinese Town

Tom McDonald

Abstract This chapter draws on ethnographic data to examine the relationship between mobile communication technologies (especially mobile phones) and learning in a small rural town in North China. Building on a wide body of literature that emphasises the enduring importance of education within Chinese culture, this chapter demonstrates how contemporary attitudes towards learning become constructed and expressed through mobile phone use. The chapter illustrates how most rural parents regard mobile phones as having an adverse impact on their offspring's academic achievement and are keen to limit their usage. Young people nevertheless continue to find ways of accessing and using mobile phones, including creatively appropriating such devices for their own (formal and informal) learning. The chapter calls for greater consideration of the multiple domains of society that such technologies cut across – including school, family and elsewhere – in order to expose the specific instances where mobile telecommunications interact with educational ideals.

Keywords China • Education • Mobile phones • Rural • Family

The shop display of the China Unicom mobile store that lay on the narrow high street of Anshan Town,[1] the small marketplace hub of a rural ward located in North China's Shandong province, differed remarkably from those found in commercial zones of large Chinese cities. While comparable mobile network outlets in nearby metropoles were replete with the latest smartphones, eager sales attendants and colourful advertising, Anshan Town's China Unicom store was a plain, dilapidated whitewashed building. The shop window of which featured a couple of lonely A3-sized advertising posters promoting a 3G SIM card package that, despite being official China Unicom marketing materials, had obviously remained in the window for such a long time so as to become faded through exposure to the strong summer sun. However, these posters were dwarfed by a two-metre-tall sign attached to the

---

[1] In order to protect the anonymity of the participants of this research, the names of all individuals, businesses and places (below city level) have been altered in this chapter.

T. McDonald (✉)
University of Hong Kong, Hong Kong, Hong Kong
e-mail: mcdonald@hku.hk

© Springer Science+Business Media Dordrecht 2016
S.S. Lim (ed.), *Mobile Communication and the Family*, Mobile Communication in Asia: Local Insights, Global Implications,
DOI 10.1007/978-94-017-7441-3_2

front of the shop, which read, in enormous white Chinese characters on an auspicious red background

> **Book Reading Youth!**
> *Electronic education.*
> *Used by experts and leaders.*
> *Reading machines.*
> *Student computers.*
> *Student tablet computers.*

Initially, it seemed senseless that the store, an official outlet of one of China's largest phone networks, should place so much emphasis on promoting these 'study machines' rather than the sale of mobile phones, when the potential market for study machines was so much smaller than that for mobile phones. Furthermore, the store made little profit from selling these machines (few of which used China Unicom's mobile network) in comparison to the 12–24-month subscription deals associated with the purchase of many mobile phones, which obliged customers to return to the store at regular intervals in order to 'top up' with extra credit.[2] However, the longer I spent in Anshan Town, the more I came to realise that the prominence that the store gave to these study machines embodied a wider set of concerns held by townsfolk, which related to the position of mobile communications within the family and their relationship with education. The advertising appeared to be motivated less by an interest in actually selling these devices and more by a desire to allay concerns that the store, by providing mobile phones and broadband internet connections,[3] was in some sense responsible for providing young people with technologies that were seen to have a detrimental effect on their academic achievement.

By examining the attitudes of local families towards mobile phones and learning, this chapter contributes to the volume by demonstrating how ideals regarding education, which is a pressing concern in Chinese society, are often evident in how mobile communications are appropriated and managed within families. In addition, by specifically focusing on mobile communications, this chapter will contribute to a more nuanced understanding of the centrality of education to Chinese life. By employing an ethnographic approach that considers how young people's actual practices of mobile phone use fit amongst the wider context of Anshan Town, it becomes possible to examine how attitudes towards education are constructed and expressed through mobile phone use. Through this methodology, the chapter aims to provide a novel perspective on how these particular technologies mediate specific desires and aspirations within the social life of families and likewise how mobile phones are used to both think through and implement such ideals.

---

[2] The standard model of mobile phone subscription in China is a hybrid contract/pay-as-you-go agreement. Subscribers pay an upfront joining fee (which may include the provision of a new handset). During the initial contract period, they receive a small monthly credit rebate alongside their data and call allowance, on the provision that their account contains sufficient credit to cover the monthly fee.

[3] Until August 2014, China Unicom was the only telecoms provider to offer broadband internet service to households within the township.

The remainder of this chapter is made up of four sections. I begin with a brief literature review, which will explain the foundations of the enduring cultural importance of education within Chinese culture, and setting this against the rapid emergence of mobile communication technologies. The second section will discuss the broad range of methodologies, ethnographic and otherwise, that were employed in order to shed light on how educational ideals interacted with mobile technologies. The third section of this chapter analyses the results of this research, discussing commonly held ideals regarding mobile phones and their perceived negative effects on the education of middle school students; aspirations and actions directed towards accessing mobile phones in the face of such discourse; and how young people in the town creatively appropriate mobile phones for their own learning. The chapter concludes by contending that an ethnographic approach to understanding mobile technology use allows consideration of the overlapping realms of society that such technologies traverse – including school, family and elsewhere – in order to uncover the specific moments where mobile telecommunications coalesce with educational ideals.

The Education and Technology Landscape

In this literature review, I first discuss a broad body of literature on the importance of education in Chinese culture, before showing how recent theoretical approaches allow for consideration of broader context and provide better frameworks for understanding the impact of mobile communication technologies on learning. The second section focuses on the growth of mobile communication technologies in China and the approaches and issues that arise.

Education in China: Considering the Broader Learning Context

Chinese society is frequently characterised as having long placed high value upon education, the acquisition of which is viewed by its members as being essential for social success (Hau and Salili 1996; Stevenson and Lee 1996). Parents feel that their children's academic accomplishment will help to ensure a comfortable life (Kipnis 2011), while also guaranteeing the latter's ability to fulfil their filial obligation to care for their parents in their old age (Stafford 2000a). Authors have noted that China's family planning policy has further increased the burden on large numbers of only children to achieve high levels of attainment (Fong 2004; Li and Li 2010).

The strong desire for education is felt in both urban and rural Chinese settings. Kipnis' (2011) ethnographic study of the education system within Zouping County, also in Shandong province, offers a convincing explanation for the strong emphasis on schooling within Chinese society. Outlining his theory of 'educational desire',

Kipnis shows how the importance that Chinese people attach to education has wide-ranging effects upon social organisation. He reports that all parents of school-age children he surveyed desired for their child to be admitted to university. He noted that this aspiration persisted despite the fact that the costs associated with university education far outweighed the short-term economic gains. While newly graduated university students typically faced bleak job prospects and low starting salaries, their peers who had chosen to obtain vocational qualifications at colleges (e.g. nursing, electrical engineering, etc.) could, upon graduation, expect to easily find a job with reasonable pay relatively. This disparity underlined how parents' wishes to send their children to university were often not based on rational economic reasoning.

Kipnis' (2011) observations regarding the emphasis the Chinese education system places on exemplary cases, whether it be 'model' teachers, students, essays, handwriting or even schools themselves, are particularly relevant here. A successful student might be one who can replicate Chinese characters with perfect form or who is able to memorise and recall large amounts of information to produce 'model' answers during examinations. This emphasis on perfectly emulating exemplars requires that students devote considerable time and effort to studying and is of particular importance in light of the explosion in mobile technologies within Chinese society, which, as this chapter will explain, is widely considered to be detrimental to academic endeavours. Notably, Kipnis' otherwise thorough ethnography largely neglects to discuss the influence of mobile phones on learning, although it was a major concern amongst my own friends in Anshan Town.

Stafford (2000b, p. 6), in his ethnography of education and child development within Chinese society,[4] rightly comments that simply claiming that 'education is important' for Chinese people constitutes a rather pedestrian statement. In contrast, he contends that 'education' ought not to be seen as a universal category. Stafford acknowledges that the rote learning and copying of Chinese characters is often viewed as being perhaps the definitive feature of Chinese education, before using his ethnography to build on claims by other anthropologists that challenge the distinction between non-formal and formal systems of learning (Borofsky 1987; Akinnaso 1992). His approach favours looking at learning as a part of life, making use of Sperber and Wilson's (1995) concept of 'drawing attention to', which holds that young people's understanding of the world is formed at key moments in everyday life when specific practices focus their attention on phenomena that are marked out as being especially important.

This chapter does not intend to focus on one definition of education at the expense of another. Rather, the aim here is to acknowledge that these contrasting definitions encompass such a broad range of activities that they make it possible to see mobile communication within the family as being related to and having an impact on education itself. Nonetheless, it ought to be acknowledged that for most people in Anshan, 'education' (*jiaoyu*) typically refers to a defined set of formal and

---

[4] Stafford's (2000b) ethnography draws on research conducted in both a Taiwanese fishing village and a village in the Heilongjiang province of north-east mainland China.

informal institutions, especially those related to schooling children and young people and that this frequently intersects with other aspects of everyday life, such as mobile phone use.

Emerging Mobile Technologies in China: Approaches and Issues

The development of mobile devices, particularly phones, has arguably been one of the key transformative agents in Chinese society in the last 15 years. The country has experienced an explosion in mobile phone ownership, with mobiles effectively leapfrogging landlines to become the *de rigeur* communication device for swathes of the population. A survey by the Pew Research Center (2014, p. 2) reported that mobile phone ownership amongst its Chinese sample (which was limited to adults and acknowledged as being 'disproportionately urban') stood at 95 %, which was the highest ownership rate of all the emerging countries in their survey. Of those sampled, 37 % reported owning a smartphone, again placing China amongst the highest of all the developing countries compared in the study. Likewise, a separate survey (Nielsen Company 2013) focusing on mobile phone usage amongst Chinese youth (between 15 and 24 years of age) recorded a smartphone ownership rate of 82 %, compared to feature phone ownership at 14 %.[5] This represents a radical transition when compared to a report published by the same company only 3 years earlier (Nielsen Company 2010), which placed smartphone usage at only 29 %, in contrast to 71 % for feature phones; however, this survey was again limited to Chinese cities. Despite the fact that the above reports largely ignore rural populations like those of Anshan Town, the figures are nonetheless significant in drawing attention to the rapidly growing importance of mobile phones (and particularly smartphones) within urban Chinese life and highlight the need to understand whether such changes are also occurring in rural China.

The extent of growth of smartphone use within China is also highlighted in a China Internet Network Information Center (CNNIC) (2014) report, which shows a dramatic year-on-year increase in the number of people in China who use mobile phones to access the internet, from 50.4 million in 2007 (24 % of total internet users) to over 500 million in 2013 (81 % of total internet users). The report also states that the number of users of the 3G mobile network reached 386 million by November 2013, which represented an increase of over 154 million compared to in the preceding 12 months.

While macro-level data such as nationally collected statistical surveys provide useful indicators of broad trends, such statistics offer little insight into how these transformations impact people's everyday lives, although there exist several theoretical models aimed at facilitating such an understanding. This chapter avoids

---

[5] The term 'feature phone' describes low-end phones with limited capabilities such as voice calls and SMS.

highly deterministic frameworks for explaining the adoption of information and communication technologies (ICTs) (Davis 1989; Rogers 1995) in favour of models that foreground the agency of individuals in appropriating technologies into their lives. One such model is the theory of technology domestication (Silverstone 1994; Silverstone and Haddon 1996; Silverstone et al. 1989, 1992), whose focus on the home and family makes it particularly apt in this chapter. An added complication though is that the use of such devices is an issue of concern for families because their portable nature means their use often occurs outside the physical confines of the house itself. Similarly, ethnographic approaches have foregrounded the importance of illustrating the specificity of the cultural contexts in which new ICTs are adopted (Miller and Slater 2000; Horst and Miller 2006).

Bray (2013) calls for a focus on human habits and practices and how they become melded with these new technologies, arguing that increased attention ought to be paid not only to technologies but especially 'to the technological repertoires associated with social roles, and to the skills and operational sequences involved in significant social activities or transactions' (p. 189), as a means to understand the moral and ethical aspects of particular economies.

Lim (2008) posits that ICTs themselves have become an important symbol of consumerism, especially in the case of mobile phones, owing to their conspicuous portability. Likewise, both Gamble (2003) and Qiu (2009) note the presence of a particular stratum of early mobile phone adopters, who made their status overt by carrying large brick-like phones (known as *dageda*) that their work units[6] purchased for them. Today, the availability of cheap domestic brands of smartphones means they have become commonplace for adults and young people throughout urban China.

Lim's (2008) research on technology domestication amongst Asian families is particularly useful in showing how consideration of mobile phone use within families can contribute to an understanding of the relationship between mobile phones and education. She observes that amongst the Beijing and Shanghai families in her study, children would frequently make use of mobile phones and MP3 players while travelling between school and home, but these items were banned within school premises. Lim also found that parents would use the phones bought for their children as 'surveillance' devices, frequently calling their children in order to establish their whereabouts, particularly as they moved between school and home. She also noted a strong parental desire to control what were felt to be diversions from education, especially ICTs that were the source of entertainment. In this way, her research focuses more on the use of the internet, computers and television by families than mobile communication technologies, as these were (at the time of Lim's fieldwork) the main conduits of entertainment. However, the enormous increase in smartphone functionality and usage within China in recent years has changed the status of the mobile phone, and therefore the information presented in this chapter is intended to

---

[6] 'Work unit' is the term used to describe the place of employment in the People's Republic of China. Qiu (2009) notes that many of the original users of *dageda* were elites employed in key work units.

contribute to a more up-to-date understanding of the mobile phone within Chinese family life.

There is a growing body of literature on how parents manage their children's ICT use. A key theme is choosing where ICTs are placed within the home (Flynn 2003; Lemor 2006; McDonald 2015), although little is written on mobile communication technologies in this regard. Lim and Soon (2010) note how management of offspring's internet use is frequently a gendered task, with mothers in many different cultural contexts tending to play a bigger role in the supervision of ICT use than fathers, while highlighting the lack of such studies in the Asian context. In this connection, and more specifically focused on mobile phones, Ito (2005) notes how Japanese mothers found it difficult to accept the private nature of their offspring's mobile use, finding it easier to simply ban their children from using mobile phones.

This literature review has focused on two opposing trends: first, the enduring importance of education within Chinese society, which is particularly apparent in the emphasis on exemplary models and examination, and second, the rapid emergence of mobile phones as one of the main communication tools within Chinese society. It is the interaction of these two trends, relatively unstudied in the context of rural China, which this chapter hopes to illuminate.

Methodology

The findings presented in this chapter stem from 15 months of ethnographic fieldwork that was conducted in Anshan Town between April 2013 and August 2014, which formed part of a larger comparative project called the Global Social Media Impact Study.[7] During the research period, I lived in a village on the edge of Anshan Town, immersing myself in the social life of the surrounding area. I was aided in this respect by my own advanced level of written and spoken Chinese and also through the prior experience of living for 18 months in a medium-sized county town in a remote part of South-west China as part of my earlier PhD research (McDonald 2013). This ethnography was combined with several more structured research/data collection methods, including extended recorded interviews, detailed questionnaires aimed at adults within the field site ($n=119$) and simplified, broader versions for young people in the local middle school ($n=312$). A follow-up questionnaire was also completed in the final month of fieldwork ($n=175$). While the original study encompassed a wide variety of persons from all age ranges, owing to space concerns, this chapter focuses only on middle school students (the town does not have a high school or a vocational college). Middle school is particularly important because achievement in the middle school examinations (*zhongkao*) dictates whether most students go on to either high school (typically leading to university) or vocational college (leading to paid employment).

---

[7] www.ucl.ac.uk/global-social-media

General ethnographic observations were recorded either in notebooks or on a computer/smartphone and subsequently developed into longer-form field notes, which were stored in a computer database to allow classification of individual notes. Face-to-face interviews were typically conducted in standard Chinese (*Putonghua*), although some respondents preferred to reply to my questions in local Shandong dialect. During the initial three months of fieldwork, I was joined by two Master's students, of Chinese nationality, from Minzu University of China in Beijing. They were able to repeat and clarify participants' responses to me in standard Chinese when I had trouble understanding. In later stages of the fieldwork, I was able to rely more on my growing knowledge of the local dialect and the help of several local research assistants. Recorded interviews were subsequently transcribed into Chinese characters remotely by a team of students in Beijing, at which point English language keywords were added to many of the responses in order to enable searching of the transcripts via computer. Questionnaire data, collected in homes, schools, workplaces and in public places, were manually inputted into a spreadsheet. This qualitative data was later subjected to further analysis using SPSS.

This approach rejects what Bernard (2006, p. viii) describes as the 'pernicious distinction' between quantitative and qualitative data. The depth of understanding that comes from ethnographic engagement and the opportunity it provides to observe specific practices of people's ICT use (see also McDonald 2015) was merged with interview data that provided insight into people's accounts of such behaviours. Statistical data was also incorporated, on the occasions when it helped to inform whether broader significance could be attached to individual practices or accounts of such practices.

Anshan Town was selected as a field site because it satisfied a number of requirements imposed by the larger comparative project of which this research is a part. The town was small in size, with official figures from 2011 placing the population of the entire township at around 32,000 and the population of the town itself at 6000.[8] Although the township is predominantly rural, there existed a small number of factories within the area that manufactured pressurised heating vessels for residential heating systems, thus providing an important stimulus to the town's economy. While by no means wealthy, the vast majority of people within the town and surrounding villages reported having experienced notable improvements in living standards since the start of the reform era and particularly during the last decade. Anshan Town's growing wealth, combined with the falling cost of smartphone and feature phone ownership, meant that for many people, possessing a mobile communication device was an affordable reality. As such, Anshan Town offered an ideal field site in which to observe how communication technologies were transforming rural Chinese family life.

---

[8] In this context 'the town' refers to the small town seat and four villages that border it, which taken together form a contiguous built-up settlement of around 0.6 square kilometres.

Discussion

The multiple intersections between mobile phones and education were observed on many occasions during fieldwork. These occasions of convergence can be separated into three main categories, which while not exhaustive, provide a useful analytical framework for understanding the main types of convergence between mobile communication and education. The first is the level of discourse, which refers to an established narrative articulated by parents (but also by significant numbers of students themselves) that focused on the negative effects of mobile phones on education. The second category, which largely acted in opposition to the anti-mobile discourse, resulted from the desires of young people to access mobile phones and their tactics – largely directed towards other family members – for realising such desires. The third aspect reflects the inventive ways in which young people *actually* used mobile phones for educational ends, some of which were plainly supportive of formal educational goals, while others, though contributing to young people's learning, were less immediately recognised by parents or students themselves as being educational. The following sections will emphasise how mobile phone purchase and use was never an entirely individual choice; rather, each of these categories shows how the whole family became implicated in issues of mobile phone appropriation, often including matters of assessing and understanding the complex relationships between mobile phones and education.

Discourse: Mobile Phones as the Antithesis of Education

The presence of an 'educational desire' (Kipnis 2011, pp. 1–2), a near-universal preference amongst Chinese parents of school-age children that their offspring would eventually attend university, was especially pronounced in Anshan Town. In addition to being expressed verbally, this thrust was also physically and institutionally manifest in multiple ways around town. Much of a child's life was spent within the classroom. In order to satisfy parents' desire for increased study time, the town's middle school offered complimentary early morning and late evening supervised 'self-study' classes outside of normal lesson times. As far as I was aware, all students regularly attended these sessions, prolonging the typical school day from 8 hours to over 14 hours (6:30 am–8:40 pm). The summer holidays provided no respite for many children, and private tuition classes (*fudao ban*) were offered in temporarily converted homes, taught by university students on vacation. Many parents seemed willing to spend considerable amounts of money on such tuition (see also Anagnost 1997).

These instances suggest that a universal educational desire similar to that described by Kipnis (2011) was felt especially strongly amongst parents of school-age children in Anshan Town. Furthermore, almost every single parent whom I spoke to throughout the course of the research believed that mobile phones (and, more broadly, the internet, gaming and social media) had an adverse effect on their child's study. This position appeared to be largely independent of any actual evidence and instead was often rooted in select anecdotal evidence based on their own experience or that of other families within the town, rather than third-party scientific assessment.

It was also clear that the widespread discourse concerning the relationship between mobile phone use and academic study was reproduced not only by parents but also by educational institutions themselves (largely staffed by teachers with children of their own), which played an active role in disseminating the assertion that mobile phones had a negative impact on educational progression. This intolerance was manifested in a number of ways, the most conspicuous and severe of which was the banning of mobile phones from school grounds. One middle school pupil explained to me that students who violated the rules by choosing to bring their phones into school could expect to have them confiscated. The manager of one of the town's private tuition schools that operated during the summer holidays provided an impassioned account of why he viewed confiscating mobile phones as a necessary deterrent:

> I taught the third grade[9] of middle school for a while. On one occasion, I confiscated five or six mobile phones. When they're using phones they're not doing anything else, just chatting on QQ,[10] reading [online short stories]... Of course, in China, students communicating with each other more is a good thing. But in China, with this kind of education for the purpose of examinations, you *must* study; communication is put in a secondary position. Because each year there is *just one chance* in the exam. If you don't pass the exam, you can only enter [manual] employment, and it will be a very bad environment, and you won't have any good way out. But in China, if you can pass the exam and get into a [good] university... then you can find some dignified work. Your salary won't be very high, but you will sit in an office, under the breeze of the air conditioning.

The teacher's account, while acknowledging the communicative potential of the mobile phone, simultaneously casts such devices as a barrier to his students' exam success, preventing them from enjoying a comfortable, safe and dignified life. Confiscation is seen as a necessary deterrent intended for the child's own benefit, so as to cultivate proper habits that facilitate effective learning.

Another middle school student explained to me that it was not uncommon for mobile phones confiscated by teachers to be withheld from the child until the end of the term or even until the end of the school year. Such measures did not appear to provoke major concern amongst parents. Instead, the school's efforts to prohibit the use of mobile phones by students not only acted in tandem with parental reservations regarding the use of mobile phones, but also reassured parents that their assertions were correct. That said, a significant minority (35 %) of phone-owning middle school children surveyed indicated that they still brought their phones to school.

---

[9] Third grade middle school students are approximately 14 years of age.
[10] QQ is a popular Chinese social networking platform. Surveys in Anshan Town indicated that for townsfolk it had the highest rate of account ownership, length of use and estimated time spent online daily of all social networks. QQ was especially popular among the town's school children.

Despite young people's desire to use and own mobile phones, the notion that mobile phones could distract from one's studies had, to a certain extent, been internalised by some young people within the town. Our survey of middle school students revealed that 64 % felt that having access to a mobile phone did indeed distract them from their study.

The draconian measure of banning mobile phones from the classroom was especially effective because school schedules, which filled close to the entirety of a student's typical week with lessons and homework, left students with extremely few instances when mobile phone use was permitted (see Table 2.1).

Table 2.1 Example of daily schedule of a second grade middle school student

Time	Activity
06:00	Get up. Brush teeth, wash face. Depart for school
06:30	Teacher supervised 'self-study' lesson
07:20	Eat breakfast, clean classroom
08:00	Class group sings song together
08:10	Lesson 1
08:55	Short break
09:05	Lesson 2
09:50	Long break
10:20	Lesson 3
11:05	Short break
11:15	Lesson 4
12:00	Return home. Lunch[a]
12:50	Return to school. Prepare for lesson
13:20	Clean classroom
13:30	Class group sings song together
13:40	Lesson 5
14:25	Short break
14:35	Lesson 6
15:20	Long break
15:50	Lesson 7
16:35	Short break
16:45	Lesson 8
17:30	Return home. Dinner[a]
18:00	Return to school. Prepare for self-study
18:30	Short break
18:40	Teacher supervised 'self-study' lesson
19:35	Short break
19:45	Teacher supervised 'self-study' lesson
20:40	School ends. Return home[a]
22:00	Sleep

[a]Denotes times when student is at home and is typically permitted to use mobile phone, computer, etc. (if available)

For example, one young male student in the third grade of middle school I spoke to told me that he owned a cheap feature phone that he used primarily for calling his mother during the lunch break. In a different example, a female student in the third grade, who lived in one of the villages in the countryside surrounding the town, explained why despite having a computer at home, she had to ask her older sister, who was in college and had a mobile phone to help maintain her online profile: 'I have no time, because I am always studying... I only have time at the weekends. During class times playing on phones isn't allowed.' Although many of the people viewing her online profile were her classmates who themselves faced similar time restrictions, a secondary motivation for staying online was that simply spending time logged in to QQ would also help to increase the ranking of her account.

In contrast to the town's middle school pupils, students attending college and university in nearby cities, such as the older sister mentioned above, were generally tacitly permitted to use mobile phones during class times. Middle and high school students complaining about the lack of opportunities to access the internet were commonplace during my fieldwork. Although it initially seemed incongruous to hear rural middle school students talking of long working hours in the manner one might expect of city bankers, nonetheless generally students took these pressures in their stride.

Perhaps most telling in relation to this discourse on the perceived negative effects of mobile phones on education were the findings from the section of the survey which asked respondents to indicate in which quartile of the class they ranked for academic results and also whether they possessed a mobile phone. It should be noted that Chinese schools frequently rank students within the same class group throughout each academic year based on examinations and assessment exercises, so most students have a fairly clear idea of how they compare to their classmates. The highest distribution of students occupied the top quartile of the class, with 29 % of all students surveyed indicating that they fell within this range (see Table 2.2).

The distribution of students decreased successively as the academic ranking of the quartiles became lower, suggesting that students with comparatively poorer results than their peers preferred to select the 'would rather not say' option than share their ranking. The roughly even distribution of students after taking into account the 'would rather not say' option suggests the self-reporting of students'

Table 2.2 Distribution of middle school students according to self-reported grade

Self-reported grade	Frequency	Per cent
Top 25 %	87	27.9
25–50 %	57	18.3
50–75 %	31	9.9
Bottom 25 %	6	1.9
'Would rather not say'	118	37.8
Missing	13	4.2
Total	**312**	**100.0**

academic position to be largely reliable. Of key interest here is the fact that when students' class position was correlated against whether they owned a mobile phone, it was discovered that there existed only marginally lower mobile phone ownership rates amongst higher-ranking school children (see Table 2.3). This suggests that, for the students sampled, claims of a correlation between mobile phone ownership and poor academic results are weak at best.

Mobile Desires vs. Educational Desires

This dominant discourse against mobile phone use in educational contexts, and the prohibitions associated with it, emerged in response to a genuine desire amongst young people in Anshan Town to be able to own and use mobile phones. This desire was motivated by a number of factors. Although some of these reasons were connected to education, many were not necessarily immediately related to academic endeavour.

As part of the questionnaire, phone-owning middle school students in Anshan Town were asked to rank their uses of their mobile phones in order of importance. The vast majority of respondents said the most important use was to access the internet (see Table 2.4). The second most important use of the mobile phone for students was as an alarm clock, reflecting the difficulty many students faced in rising for the 6:30 am start of the school day. The least important functions of the mobile phone, according to the students, were sending traditional text messages (now largely replaced by a combination of QQ Instant Messenger and WeChat) and studying.

Students in Anshan Town adopted a wide range of strategies to increase opportunities for Internet use, especially via mobile phones. Although broadband service was available throughout most of the township, including in more remote villages, according to informal conversation with the manager of the town's China Unicom store, only around one-third of households had it installed. This was largely due to the fact that 610 RMB (approximately US$99) annual broadband subscription[11] was

Table 2.3 Cross tabulation between self-reported grade of middle school students and phone ownership

Self-reported grade	Phone ownership (per cent)		Total share (per cent)
	Own	Do not own	
Top 25 %	25.7	33.9	29.3
25–50 %	17.4	20.5	18.7
50–75 %	13.2	7.1	10.5
Bottom 25 %	2.4	1.6	2.0
'Would rather not say'	41.3	37.0	39.5
Total	**100**	**100**	**100**

n = 294

---

[11] Price correct as of May 2013

Table 2.4 Responses to question, 'what is the main use of your mobile phone?'

Main use	Frequency
Internet	105
Alarm clock	84
Calling	65
Texting	31
Studying	31

judged to be an unnecessary expense by most families. In contrast, many (predominantly male) household heads viewed the purchase of a 3G smartphone as a legitimate expense, even if they themselves did not typically use the internet.

The ownership of these mobile phones within households by parents or adult siblings offered many young people in the town the opportunity to access the internet, with some 40 % of middle school students reporting accessing the internet mainly through mobile phones. One such student was a young girl from the third grade. Her father prohibited her from owning a mobile phone, and as the family did not have a broadband connection in their home, her main method of accessing the internet was by borrowing her father's phone and 'helping him to use the bandwidth' (*bang ta yong liuliang*). This refers to the fact that most mobile subscriptions include a set amount of free calls and bandwidth; however, it is typically the case that middle-aged people prefer making telephone calls to using the internet and hence use little (if any) bandwidth. In this way, young people's 'help' serves as a justification for their internet access, made under the pretext of optimising their parents' excess resources, thereby yielding greater value from their expenses.

Educational Ingenuity

While acknowledging that the majority of mobile phone use amongst the young people of Anshan Town appeared to have little to do with education, there remained instances where young people's appropriation of mobile phones did contribute, in various ways, to their learning. One of the key findings in this regard concerns the way in which students use mobile phones, and more specifically the social media that can be accessed through them, as a means to prolong and expand the social groupings that are created by schools themselves and to transcend the spatial confines of the school. Central to this is how communication between classmates dominate students' patterns of mobile phone use, and the class group (*ban*) is of particular importance in this respect. A normal class group in Anshan Town's middle school would typically remain in the same physical classroom for most of the day, with teachers moving between classrooms, and remarkably few occasions in which students were made to work together with parties other than the class group. In sum, the class group appears to be a group of people who often became the basis of enduring friendships. Indeed, I often witnessed 'class group reunions' in the town, where former classmates who were now in their twenties or thirties would meet in order to eat together and socialise.

Access to the internet via mobile phones (and to a lesser extent, via home broadband connections) has provided students with the opportunity to reproduce the classmate group within another space. This is most apparent in the case of 'QQ groups'. QQ includes an instant messaging client that is used throughout China, and although its popularity appears to have waned somewhat with the advent of other social media platforms in the country (i.e. WeChat, Weibo), it remains the main social media platform within Anshan Town and is especially popular amongst school-age children. QQ groups permit users to create ongoing instant messaging conversations amongst a defined (and usually closed) group of users, of which some have administrator roles and the ability to add or remove other members. School-age children appear to be very keen to establish these groups, a large number of which are based around class groups, with students asking their classmates to join the group during classes or via direct instant message. The groups are often named after the members' class group number. Several students commented that it was not uncommon for a single class group to have several QQ groups, each set up by a different student, who would act as 'group owner' (*qun zhuren*) for the group in question and was also able to appoint group administrators (*guanli yuan*). In effect, these groups seemed to be vying with one another for popularity.

Several students shared that they found the constant messages between the group administrator and their close friends to be especially irritating (*fan*). However, they did not wish to leave the group for fear that their classmates would take offence. Many explained that they felt the best solution in such a situation was to 'silence' (*pingbi*) the group so that they remained a member but did not receive notifications when new messages were posted. Green and Haddon's (2009, pp. 101–105) concept of the 'management of availability' as being of key import in mobile communications is useful here. The authors highlight the popular understanding that 'communicative access to others anytime and anywhere' offered by the mobile phone is seen as 'both desirable and beneficial'. Instead, people practise a process of 'selective sociality' (Fortunati 2002; Matsuda 2005) managing when and with whom one is available for access.

Despite such annoyances, a significant number of students still felt these QQ groups were useful in that they gave students a forum in which to discuss school-related matters outside of the school itself, although it should be noted that such discussions seemed to form only a minor part of the overall use of QQ groups. These groups were also important in a further sense – many of them continued to provide forums for communication after students graduated from school whereupon the class group ceased to meet regularly.

One aspect of class group-based QQ groups that several students also highlighted as being of importance was their role in facilitating the completion of homework assignments. Much of the homework that students were assigned was in the form of take-home papers, most of which comprised numbered questions with multiple-choice or single-word answers. On several occasions, I observed students in their homes obtaining the answers from each other by exchanging messages within the class group-based QQ groups. Students forming their own informal online homework help groups made sense given that many rural parents had only received primary or middle school education and thus often found it difficult to help their children with homework. Thus, QQ groups helped students to access a wider network of support.

Another significant implication of the fact that students' activities on mobile phones occurred out of sight of both teachers and parents was that it gave these young people an increased opportunity to chat with each other and this proved central to establishing romantic relationships. Schools prohibited romantic associations between classmates for fear that such relations, like mobile phones themselves, would adversely affect students' study. Most parents also shared the view that relationships amongst school-age students were problematic. Mobile telecommunications provided a way for young people to engage in romantic relationships that were intimate and yet maintained the physical distance necessary to avoid detection by parents and teachers. One high school student in Anshan Town told me that he had several different QQ accounts, some of which his parents did not know the password for, so that he was able to chat with girls online without his parents' knowledge. It was (readily) apparent that, faced with these restrictions, students saw mobile phones as a means to speak directly to potential romantic partners without others finding out.

A final noteworthy aspect of young people's appropriation of mobile phones that ought to be considered as educational is that knowing how to use these devices was becoming increasingly important for creating and maintaining social relations. This was especially so for poorer households in the outlying countryside where broadband internet connections at home were rare and only limited time was given over to access in school. In such cases, mobile phones constituted an important avenue for learning and experimenting with the digital skills that have become steadily more indispensable in contemporary Chinese society.

In this section, I have deliberately chosen a loose, anthropological definition of education that extends beyond formal schooling (although some of the strategies discussed above are instructive in this regard) to include the learning and utilisation of social and cultural conventions. This deliberately broad interpretation of education permits consideration of a more wide-ranging set of implications associated with young people's phone use. In this context, it ought also to be emphasised that the educational uses of mobile phones listed here do not necessarily imply that the students exhibit such defined educational 'intentionality' while using phones. While some practices appear to be clearly linked to learning, with others the connection is somewhat more tenuous. What all of these different behaviours have in common, however, is that they demonstrate young people's ingenuity in appropriating mobile phones for their own ends.

Conclusion: Understanding Education through Mobile Phones

The data presented above illustrate specific ways in which the almost universal educational desire that Kipnis (2011) claimed to be a distinctive feature of Chinese society finds expression in relation to new technologies, such as mobile phones, entering into family life. The discussions expand Kipnis' understanding of educational desire by showing how it can be constituted through an incredibly wide array of objects and phenomena, including mobile communication technologies.

Furthermore, this chapter has demonstrated the tendency for people's attitudes towards ICTs to be informed by their generational position within families. The data revealed a widely held belief amongst parents of school-age children that the latter's use of mobile phones has an adverse effect on their study. Furthermore, a smaller (although still significant) proportion of school-age children themselves believed mobile phones were an obstacle to their own educational attainment.

Universal educational desire was compared to the desire for mobile phones amongst young people in the field site, where young people employed a number of strategies either to gain temporary access to phones (through borrowing, etc.) or to persuade their parents to gift them phones outright.

The final section of this chapter concentrated on the ways in which phones were actually used for educational purposes by young people, most of which were discerned through ethnographic observation. These included replicating the class group unit outside of school through the use of QQ groups, using mobile phones to engage in prohibited romantic relationships and the acquisition of digital skills.

One of the key conclusions that can be drawn from these three different aspects of mobile phone use is that these technologies have a broad, and often unforeseen, range of impacts. Making moralistic judgements about the consumption of particular technologies does not get one closer to understanding the actual use and effects of such technologies in people's lives (Miller 2001). Likewise, the findings presented in this paper complicate the prevalent discourse, evident amongst both Anshan Town adults and more broadly in academic writing, that mobile phones and other new communication technologies necessarily have a negative influence on productivity or diminish our humanity (Turkle 2011). By examining young people's desires for mobile phones, the techniques and strategies employed to gain access to such devices and the inventive ways in which they appropriate mobile phones for educational ends, one comes to see mobile phones in a different light: as a point around which families understand, construct and enact desires for educational achievement for their school-age children.

Such an approach, which holds that mobile phones are not merely a communication device but also a locus around which ideas and concepts of personal achievement, good parenting and social relationships coalesce, can also help cement a move away from analysis of these ICTs within techno-deterministic or functionalistic frameworks (Davis 1989; Rogers 1995), in favour of approaches that focus on the social characteristics of these technologies (Silverstone et al. 1992) and what they *actually* mean to the people who *actually* use them. Furthermore, the portability of mobile communication technologies makes them especially important for social sciences research, as their ability to be moved with ease tends to involve them in wider networks of social relations – such as schools or peer groups – than other ICTs which may be confined to the domestic sphere and can help to challenge bounded concepts of 'home' or 'family'. This makes thinking through these mobile technologies all the more important, as through them it becomes possible to gain insight into the aspirations, relationships and networks that underlie contemporary rural Chinese families.

Acknowledgements I am incredibly grateful to Elisabetta Costa, Nell Haynes, Daniel Miller, David Jobanputra, Razvan Nicolescu, Jolynna Sinanan, Juliano Spyer, Shriram Venkatraman, Sun Sun Lim and Xinyuan Wang who provided extensive comments on several draft versions of this chapter. I am particularly grateful to Ying Zhang, Zhixian Liu and Yinxue Li from Minzu University of China for their support throughout the fieldwork period. Thanks must go to the people of Anshan Town, especially the staff and students of the town's middle school for their eagerness to help with this project. This research was funded by the European Research Council (ERC Project 2011-AdG-295486 SocNet).

References

Akinnaso, F. N. (1992). Schooling, language and knowledge in literate and nonliterate societies. *Comparative Studies in Society and History, 34*(1), 68–109.
Anagnost, A. (1997). Children and national transcendence in China. In K. G. Lieberthal, S. F. Lim, & E. P. Young (Eds.), *Constructing China: The interaction of culture and economics* (pp. 195–222). Ann Arbour: Centre for Chinese Studies, University of Michigan.
Bernard, H. R. (2006). *Research methods in anthropology: Qualitative and quantitative approaches* (4th ed.). Oxford: AltaMira Press.
Borofsky, R. (1987). *Making history: Pukapukan and anthropological constructions of knowledge*. Cambridge: Cambridge University Press.
Bray, F. (2013). Tools for virtuous action: Technology, skills and ordinary ethics. In C. Stafford (Ed.), *Ordinary ethics in China* (pp. 175–193). London: Bloomsbury.
China Internet Network Information Center (CNNIC). (2014). Statistical report on internet development in China. http://www1.cnnic.cn/IDR/ReportDownloads/201404/U020140417607531610855.pdf Accessed 20 Oct 2012.
Davis, F. D. (1989). Perceived usefulness, perceived ease of use, and user acceptance of information technology. *MIS Quarterly, 13*, 319–340.
Flynn, B. (2003). Geography of the digital hearth. *Information, Communication and Society, 6*(4), 551–576.
Fong, V. L. (2004). *Only hope: Coming of age under China's one-child policy*. Stanford: Stanford University Press.
Fortunati, L. (2002). Italy: Stereotypes, true and false. In J. E. Katz & M. A. Aakhus (Eds.), *Perpetual contact: Mobile communication, private talk, public performance* (pp. 42–62). Cambridge: Cambridge University Press.
Gamble, J. (2003). *Shanghai in transition: Changing perspectives and social contours of a Chinese metropolis*. London: Routledge.
Green, N., & Haddon, L. (2009). *Mobile communications: An introduction to new media*. Oxford: Berg.

Hau, K. T., & Salili, F. (1996). Achievement goals and causal attributions of Chinese students. In S. Lau (Ed.), *Growing up the Chinese way* (pp. 121–146). Hong Kong: The Chinese University Press.

Horst, H. A., & Miller, D. (2006). *The cell phone: An anthropology of communication*. Oxford/New York: Berg.

Ito, M. (2005). Mobile phones, Japanese youth, and the re-placement of social contact. In R. Ling & P. E. Pedersen (Eds.), *Mobile communications: Renegotiation of the social sphere* (pp. 131–148). London: Springer.

Kipnis, A. B. (2011). *Governing educational desire: Culture, politics, and schooling in China*. Chicago: University of Chicago Press.

Lemor, A. M. R. (2006). Making a "home". The domestication of information and communication technologies in single mothers' households. In T. Berker, M. Hartmann, Y. Punie, & K. Ward (Eds.), *Domestication of media and technologies* (pp. 165–181). Maidenhead: Open University Press.

Li, W., & Li, Y. (2010). An analysis on social and cultural background of the resistance for China's education reform and academic pressure. *International Education Studies, 3*(3), 211–215.

Lim, S. S. (2008). Technology domestication in the Asian homestead: Comparing the experiences of middle class families in China and South Korea. *East Asian Science, Technology and Society, 2*(2), 189–209.

Lim, S. S., & Soon, C. (2010). The influence of social and cultural factors on mothers' domestication of household ICTs – Experiences of Chinese and Korean women. *Telematics and Informatics, 27*(3), 205–216.

Matsuda, M. (2005). Mobile communication and selective sociality. In M. Ito, D. Okabe, & M. Matsuda (Eds.), *Personal, portable, pedestrian: Mobile phones in Japanese life* (pp. 123–142). Cambridge, MA/London: MIT Press

McDonald, T. N. (2013). *Structures of hosting in a south-western Chinese town*. Doctoral dissertation, UCL (University College London).

McDonald, T. (2015). Affecting relations: Domesticating the internet in a south-western Chinese town. *Information, Communication & Society, 18*(1), 17–31.

Miller, D. (2001). The poverty of morality. *Journal of Consumer Culture, 1*(2), 225–243.

Miller, D., & Slater, D. (2000). *The internet: An ethnographic approach*. Oxford: Berg.

Nielsen Company. (2010). Mobile youth around the world. Retrieved from http://www.nielsen.com/content/dam/corporate/us/en/reports-downloads/2010-Reports/Nielsen-Mobile-Youth-Around-The-World-Dec-2010.pdf

Nielsen Company. (2013). The mobile consumer: A global snapshot. Retrieved from http://www.nielsen.com/content/dam/corporate/us/en/reports-downloads/2013%20Reports/Mobile-Consumer-Report-2013.pdf

Pew Research Center. (2014). Emerging nations embrace internet, mobile technology. Retrieved from http://www.pewglobal.org/files/2014/02/Pew-Research-Center-Global-Attitudes-Project-Technology-Report-FINAL-February-13-20146.pdf

Qiu, J. L. (2009). *Working-class network society: Communication technology and the information have-less in urban China*. Cambridge, MA: The MIT Press.

Rogers, E. M. (1995). *Diffusion of innovations*. New York: Free Press.

Silverstone, R. (1994). *Television and everyday life*. London: Routledge.

Silverstone, R., & Haddon, L. (1996). Design and the domestication of information and communication technologies: Technical change and everyday life. In R. Silverstone & R. Mansell (Eds.), *Communication by design: The politics of information and communication technologies* (pp. 44–74). Oxford: Oxford University Press.

Silverstone, R., Morley, D., Dahlberg, A., & Livingstone, S. (1989). *Families, technologies and consumption: The household and information and communication technologies*. CRICT discussion paper. Uxbridge: Centre for Research into Innovation, Culture & Technology.

Silverstone, R., Hirsch, E., & Morley, D. (1992). Information and communication technologies and the moral economy of the household. In R. Silverstone & E. Hirsch (Eds.), *Consuming technologies: Media and information in domestic spaces* (pp. 15–31). London: Routledge.

Sperber, D., & Wilson, D. (1995). *Relevance: Communication and cognition.* Oxford: Blackwell.

Stafford, C. (2000a). Chinese patriliny and the cycles of Yang and Laiwang. In J. Carsten (Ed.), *Cultures of relatedness: New approaches to the study of kinship* (pp. 37–54). Cambridge: Cambridge University Press.

Stafford, C. (2000b). *Separation and reunion in modern China.* Cambridge: Cambridge University Press.

Stevenson, H. W., & Lee, S.-Y. (1996). The academic achievement of Chinese students. In M. H. Bond (Ed.), *The handbook of Chinese psychology* (pp. 124–142). Hong Kong: Oxford University Press.

Turkle, S. (2011). *Alone together: Why we expect more from technology and less from each other.* New York: Basic Books.

Chapter 3
Balancing Religion, Technology and Parenthood: Indonesian Muslim Mothers' Supervision of Children's Internet Use

Rahayu and Sun Sun Lim

Abstract As technology adoption accelerates in Indonesia, the growing use of the internet by children has triggered moral panics and led to calls for greater parental mediation of children's internet use. Concerns typically center around access to online pornography and other deleterious content. The polemic surrounding these issues has taken on a distinctly moralistic and religious tone in this predominantly Muslim country. Cultural and ideological norms in Indonesia dictate that within the household, mothers are to play a key role in the supervision of children, thus placing them at the forefront of this drive to inculcate positive internet use amongst their children. This study used in-depth interviews to explore the perceptions that Indonesian Muslim mothers have of the internet, the strategies they employ to mediate the internet for their children and how their religious beliefs influence these strategies. We found that mothers actively manage their children's internet consumption and devise different mediation strategies to ensure that their children use the internet in ways that are congruent with Islamic principles. The more religious families strive to strengthen their faiths to meet the onslaught of un-Islamic internet and media content, while less devout Muslims see online media as beneficial and horizon broadening and therefore welcome rather than resist them.

Keywords Religion • Internet • Indonesia • Islam • Mothers • Parental mediation

---

Rahayu (✉)
Gadjah Mada University, Yogyakarta, Indonesia
e-mail: rahayu@ugm.ac.id

S.S. Lim
Department of Communications and New Media,
National University of Singapore, Singapore
e-mail: sunlim@nus.edu.sg

Introduction

The ascent of technology within Indonesia as its economy develops has been rapid. The internet, in particular, has made its presence felt in Indonesia's changing media landscape. Among Indonesian children, in particular, emerging research shows that they spend 2 hours a day accessing the internet. Their favourite online activities include online gaming and browsing for information. The growing use (and abuse) of the internet by Indonesian children has stoked debate within the country about the need for greater parental mediation of children's internet use, with concerns centring around access to online pornography and other deleterious content. Given that Indonesia is a predominantly Muslim country, it is not surprising that the polemic surrounding these issues has taken on a distinctly moralistic and religious tone. Cultural and ideological norms in Indonesia dictate that within the household, mothers are to play a key role in the supervision of children, thus placing Indonesian women at the forefront of this drive to inculcate positive internet use in Indonesian children. This study seeks to understand the perceptions Indonesian Muslim mothers hold regarding the internet, the strategies they employ to mediate the internet for their children and how their religious beliefs influence these strategies. We also consider how they balance their religious ideals with the practical realities of parenting in an era where technologies such as the internet are seen as inevitable. The chapter begins with a review of the growing concerns in Indonesia surrounding children's internet use, in the wake of rising adoption of the medium. We then shift our focus towards religious perceptions of the internet as held by Indonesia's Muslim community. Thereafter, we situate our study within extant literature on parental mediation of children's media use, before proceeding to explain our research method and discussing our key findings.

Indonesia's Evolving Media Landscape

The fall of Suharto in 1998 was the beginning of a new era in Indonesia. Called *Reformasi*, this political shift also ushered in dramatic changes in the media landscape resulting from the democratisation and liberalisation of the media industry (Kitley 2000; Sen and Hill 2007; Hidayat 2003). This transformation also stimulated the increase in internet usage. As of 2013, 7.5 % of all tweets globally originate from Indonesia making it the third largest Twitter country and 92.9 % of the country's internet population is using Facebook (On Device Research 2013). These trends are likely to rise further in light of the Indonesian government's policy to accelerate the utilisation of information and communication technology (ICT) in Indonesia.

On the domestic front, households with children have been similarly caught up in the internet wave. Recent studies show that most Indonesian children access the internet from home for about 2 hours a day, with internet cafés and schools being alternative sites of access (Nur 2011; Sarwono et al. 2011). They use the internet mostly for online gaming, researching school projects, chatting, email and downloading media content. Notably, these studies also suggest that many children access the internet unsupervised and that their parents do not impose any rules or supervision. Some children confessed to having viewed pornographic content and also have their own Facebook accounts even though they were underaged. The growing use of the internet by Indonesian children has raised concerns about their exposure to unsavoury or frivolous content that contains excessive sex, violence, mysticism and hedonism, and their potentially deleterious effects. Such apprehensions have been reflected in demands for the state to more actively regulate the internet and to introduce media literacy education in a more systematic and comprehensive manner. In 2010, just a day before Ramadan, the Indonesian Ministry of Communication and Informatics responded to this public pressure. It first instructed the biggest six ISPs (Indosat, Indosat Mega Media, XL Axiata, Telkomsel, Bakrie Telecom and PT Telkom), and subsequently other providers, to block access to pornographic content on the internet. However, this blanket move incited public criticism. The ministry then took a different approach to pornographic content, introducing an internet literacy program entitled '*internet Sehat dan internet Aman*' (Healthy and Safe internet), to apprise young people about how to use the internet in a more positive manner. Some schools were also provided with internet filtering software to prevent access to online pornographic content within the school environment.

Islamic Perceptions of the Internet

With Islam being Indonesia's dominant religion, practised by 88.22 % of the population (Indonesia-Investments n.d.-a), it is not surprising that compared to Indonesians of other faiths, the Islamic community has been far more vocal and fervent in its criticism of media content. As Stout (2001) noted, Islamic criticisms of the media stem from the perceptions that messages contained within popular media conflict with Islam's moral beliefs and contradict Islamic values. In particular, pornographic content online and in mainstream media are believed to cause a decline in Islamic devotees' moral and religious commitment (Fealy and White 2008). Furthermore, Western media is believed to propagate prejudicial representations of Islam and Muslims that discredit the religion and undermine its global standing (Mir-Hosseini 1998).

Despite these reservations about media content and their dissemination platforms, i.e., print and broadcast media, the internet, and mobile media devices, etc., Indonesian Muslims have been enthusiastic adopters of the internet and other forms of new media such as the mobile phone (Fealy and White 2008). Some Indonesian *da'i* (preachers) use the internet and mobile phone text messages to improve the effectiveness of their *dakwah* (preaching) and to deliver religious services. In addition, some Islamic schools have developed internet e-learning applications to socialise teachers and students on the central tenets of their faith. Such examples instantiate Stout's (2001, p. 9) claim that Muslims 'create variations in the ways popular culture is defined and used'.

Within the Islamic community, there are differing opinions on how media content should be regulated. With regard to the internet in particular, radical and extremist Islamic groups such as *Laskar Jihad* (Jihad Brigade) and *Front Pembela Islam* (Islamic Defense Front) argue that the Indonesian government and internet service providers should impose strictly enforced bans on pornographic websites. In contrast, other Islamic groups, such as *Muhammadiyah* (the second largest Muslim organisation in Indonesia), prefer to regulate the internet and its users within the private realm of the household. *Aisyiyah*, *Muhammadiyah's* women's wing, prefers to campaign for media literacy education in schools and Islamic study groups in order to empower internet users to be critical of the medium (Nur 2011), using the *Qur'an* and *Hadith* (a report of the words and deeds of the Prophet Muhammad transmitted through a chain of narrators) as the basis for such educational initiatives. Normative expectations, cultural, ideological or otherwise, make Indonesian mothers natural targets of media literacy campaigns in Indonesia (e.g. Fadhal et al. 2011; Guntarto 2011; Nur 2011), as the supervision of children is considered to be their key role in society. Furthermore, the family is considered a pillar for developing Islamic society, and Muslim women are seen as playing a crucial role in the family as the 'guide keeper' to socialise children on Islamic beliefs and values (Ida 2009).

Muslim Women's Position in Indonesian Society

To better apprehend the burdens placed on Indonesian Muslim mothers vis-à-vis parental mediation of their children's media use, we need to consider their position in Indonesian society and within Muslim households. Although in the last few decades, the number of Indonesian women participating in the labour force has risen (Indonesia-Investments n.d.-b) and perceptions of women have changed to some extent, women are still expected to serve mainly in the domestic realm (Ida 2009). Two dominant yet opposing views of women's position in Indonesian society prevail. On the one hand, women are perceived as being of inferior status to men, thereby relegating them to playing purely domestic roles. Conversely, women are viewed as being equal to men, in which women are deemed capable of performing professional and public duties. Before *Reformasi*, especially under Suharto's New Order regime, the role of women in Indonesian society was determined in the context of national development goals (Oey-Gardiner 2002; Ida 2009). "Women were assigned the role of their *kodrat* (inherent nature) and were responsible for household matters, reproduction, and family nurturing" (Ida 2009, p. 15). Even though women were identified in development programs as equal partners of men and have also worked outside the home, their position in society continues to be constrained by patriarchal ideas about women's nature, dignity and status (Ida 2009, p. 16). After *Reformasi*, the position of women in Indonesian society began to challenge the traditional model of patriarchal domination. In this new era, sociopolitical and economic changes have encouraged Indonesian women to gain access to education and to enter the workforce and political arena (Ida 2009). However, many women still face a dilemma between their 'domestic' and 'public' roles and their efforts to balance the two (Sudarto 2008; Subiantoro 2008).

Beyond broader societal conceptions, Islamic values also prescribe and proscribe vis-à-vis the status and role of Indonesian Muslim women. Competing interpretations of the *Qur'an*, *Hadith* and *Fiqh* (Islamic jurisprudence that involves the interpretation of the *Qur'an* and *Hadith*) have ignited debates (see in Van Doorn-Harder 2002; Bano 2003), with some believing that women should be confined to domestic tasks, while others feel that women can play constructive roles in the public realm. Nevertheless, new trends in the interpretations of the *Qur'an* on gender issues have brought about an advancement of women's positions in Islamic society (see in Stowasser 1998; Kazmi 1994), and women are entrusted with *socialising* children on Islamic beliefs and values.

Mothers' Roles in Parental Mediation of ICT Use

Studies of mothers and their involvement in managing household ICT use in various contexts have shown that mothers utilise media to support their parental obligations. For example, Dutch mothers improve their internet skills in order to help their children excel in school (Hynes and Rommes 2006). Similarly, mothers in Australia recognise the usefulness of the internet when they assist their children in homework (Singh 2001). Nonetheless, even though mothers recognise the value of adopting and domesticating ICTs, they may not have the authority to decide on the household's ICT purchases. In some contexts, these decisions are made based on traditional family role structures. For example, in Korea, the decision-making on products meant for family use, such as computers, is primarily dominated by men (Na et al. 1998; Na 2001).

Social expectations and cultural conventions still have bearing on women's status and position in society (Rakow and Navarro 1993; Kulik 2004; Frissen 2000). Although employment opportunities for women and the size of the female workforce are increasing, women still bear the brunt of domestic responsibilities such as managing domestic chores and childcare. This prevailing trend determines the role which women play in domesticating household ICTs and in supervising the children's use of the same. Mothers tend to be more involved than fathers in supervising their children's ICT use (Singh 2001; Anderson and Shrum 2007; Na 2001; Dholakia 2006; Pasquier 2001; Rakow and Navarro 1993; Ribak 2001). Other studies have also found that mothers have more control than fathers over where media are placed in the house in order to maximise their utility (e.g. Flynn 2003; Lemor 2006).

Parental mediation of children's media use is far from homogeneous, and several studies have attempted to identify various mediation styles. Extant research seems to centre around three identified styles: (i) restrictive mediation (rule-making such as setting the duration of media access, prohibiting access to particular content genres and restricting the location of media use) (e.g. Bybee et al. 1982; Weaver and Barbour 1992; Valkenburg Krcmar et al. 1999); (ii) active mediation (parents discuss media content with their children) (e.g. Austin 1993; Austin et al. 1990), also referred to as instructive mediation and evaluative mediation because it includes parental rationalisations and critiques of media content (e.g. Bybee et al. 1982; Messaris 1982; Valkenburg et al. 1999); and (iii) co-viewing (in which parents and children access media together and share the viewing experience but do not intentionally focus on discussing a particular program or content type) (e.g. Dorr et al. 1989; Valkenburg et al. 1999). Within the Indonesian context, scholars have observed a similar variety of parental mediation practices, with evidence for some diversionary approaches being used, e.g. some parents ask their children to play with friends and attend tuition classes and *Qur'an* education schools so as to channel their children's attention away from media (Sarwono et al. 2011).

Extant literature on other countries also indicates that the socio-economic status of parents influences parental mediation styles. Parents with media experience have a strong preference for co-viewing and active mediation, while parents with little or no experience tend to apply restrictive mediation (Bull 2005). Parents with a negative attitude towards media prefer active and restrictive mediation, whereas parents with a positive attitude prefer to engage in co-viewing (Nathanson 2001). Most middle-class families with media-rich homes tend to apply more extensive mediation and to combine multiple styles of supervision when compared to lower SES families (Notten and Kraaykamp 2009; Livingstone and Helsper 2008). Parents who are in full-time employment are less likely to set media-viewing rules, while single parents are more likely to employ co-viewing (Lin and Atkin 1989). On their part, educated parents are more likely to apply restrictive and instructive mediation (Valkenburg et al. 1999). Families staying in urban areas are more likely to engage in instructive as well as restrictive mediation than families in rural areas which tend to apply more co-viewing (Sun 2009). Besides the attributes of parents and households, children's attributes such as gender, age, school grade, and media habit have also been predicted to influence the style of parental mediation (Lin and Atkin 1989; Abanto 2004; Bybee et al. 1982; Gentile et al. 2007).

Besides demographic characteristics, religious beliefs also influence parental mediation, as some studies show. Most prior research about religion and the media have examined the influence of religious beliefs on media usage (e.g. Hamilton and Rubin 1992; Armfield and Holbert 2003; Alters 2004; Croucher et al. 2010; Golan and Day 2010). However, research specifically focusing on how religious beliefs affect parental mediation is still limited. Islam has received little attention on this front, as such research often focuses on religions such as Christianity, and other religions besides Islam (Stout and Buddenbaum 1996). One notable exception is Clark's study (2004) of a Muslim family, in North America, which applied very restrictive rules about media use on their children, seeking to instill a perceptible distance between their religious and cultural background and US culture.

The few studies which focused on the media use of Muslims have mostly been undertaken in developed Western countries such as the US (e.g. Clark 2004), Britain (e.g. Croucher et al. 2010) and France (e.g. Croucher et al. 2009) rather than in developing Asian countries such as Indonesia. This provides the present study with a research opportunity because even though Muslims worldwide are guided in their religious practice by the *Qur'an* and *Hadith*, societal structures and Islamic practices differ from country to country. Islam's development in Indonesia cannot be separated from the religion's global trends or divorced from the process of acculturation between Islam and Indonesia's indigenous cultures. Indonesia's brand of Islam is therefore distinct from those of other countries such as those in the Arab world (Wanandi 2002). Hence, the unique traits of Islamic practice in Indonesia as well as social norms surrounding the position and role of Muslim women in Indonesian society should be borne in mind when exploring the influence of religious beliefs on parental mediation of children's media use by Indonesian mothers.

In light of prior research and the overarching goals of our study, this chapter explores the following questions:

1. Do Indonesian mothers' religious beliefs shape their perceptions of the risks and opportunities of the internet, and if so, in what ways?
2. Do their religious beliefs influence the mediation strategies they apply to their children's internet use, and if so, how?
3. How do the mothers balance their religious ideals with the practical exigencies of parental mediation?

Methodology

To meet the research goals of the present study, we adopted ethnographic interviews to obtain in-depth insights articulated from a native point of view, within a natural setting. We interviewed 70 informants who met the following criteria: (1) Muslim mothers who hold Yogyakarta residents' identity card, (2) have at least one child aged 8–10 years, (3) have internet access at home, and (4) allow their children to use the internet. The recruitment of informants was launched through the first author's personal contacts and then continued via snowballing techniques. Another channel of recruitment was through members of *Aisyiyah*. Potential informants were contacted by email or voice calls which explained to them the nature of the present study and its purpose. After which, they were also sent a letter of invitation to participate in the research. Ten local research assistants were hired to facilitate the recruitment process and to conduct the interviews. All the research assistants were hired on the basis of their prior experience in conducting interviews and were also asked to undergo a 7-hour training program which apprised them of the study's research goals and processes.

This research was conducted in *Kodya Yogyakarta* in the Province of DI Yogyakarta-Indonesia for the following reasons. In this city, Muslims are dominant, constituting 90.31 % of the total population 951,611 (BPS-Statistic of D.I. Yogyakarta Province 2010), and the beliefs of Yogyakarta residents have been strongly influenced by the *Muhammadiyah* doctrine. *Muhammadiyah* is regarded as a reformist organisation because of its movement to purify Indonesian Islam from *syncretism*, a traditional theology which combines animism and Hindu–Buddhist values. *Muhammadiyah's* doctrine is based predominantly on the *Qur'an* and *Hadith* as the supreme authorities of Islamic law (Peacock 1978).

In this study, 66 of our informants stated that they are followers of *Muhammadiyah* and 20 of them are active in the board of this organisation, especially *Aisyiyah*. Forty-four also regularly attend *Qur'an* study groups and Islamic group gatherings such as preaching sessions at least once a month. Only five informants said that they were not involved in any religious activities because they were too busy with their daily activities and one informant expressed a complete lack of interest. Table 3.1 below presents the broad profile of our informants.

Table 3.1 Overview of attributes of informants

No.	Attributes of informant	Frequency
1.	Education:	
	(a) Graduated from a university (Diploma)	5
	(b) Graduated from a university (BA)	38
	(c) Graduates from a university (MA)	3
	(d) Finished high school	18
	(e) Finished primary and secondary school	4
	(f) Others (no information)	2
2.	Occupation:	
	(a) Full-time employment	37
	(b) Self-employed (in home-based businesses)	17
	(c) Homemaker	13
	(d) Others (no information)	3
3.	Number of children:	
	(a) One child	8
	(b) Two children	32
	(c) Three children	22
	(d) More than three (four and five children)	8
4.	Age:	
	(a) 25–30 years old	1
	(b) 31–36 years old	15
	(c) 37–42 years old	27
	(d) 43–48 years old	15
	(e) Above 48 years old (50 years old)	1
	(f) Others (no information)	11
5.	Internet access at home:	
	(a) ≤ 1 year	11
	(b) 1–<3 years	26
	(c) 3–<5 years	12
	(d) ≤ 5 years and above	11
	(e) Others (no information)	10

The location of the interviews was each informant's home because it is the site of daily family life where parental mediation practices are exercised (Bakardjieva and Smith 2001). However, at the request of some informants, some interviews were held at mutually agreed upon venues that were close to their homes. Each interview was conducted in the native Indonesian language (*Bahasa Indonesia*), lasted between 60 and 120 minutes and was audio-recorded. The research procedure included two activities: First, a semistructured interview where informants were asked questions about their values, beliefs and perceptions of media, not only specifically about the internet but also about the media in general. They were also asked to share their experiences of their media use and their parental mediation practices. Second, photographs were taken of the computer–internet space in the informants' homes to get a sense of where the family places different media devices. A sketch of the house was also made to describe the location and function of different rooms.

All the interviews were transcribed into *Bahasa Indonesia*, with selected quotes reported in the present chapter translated into English. Data analysis was conducted using the 'meaning condensation' approach (Kvale 1996). In this analysis, transcripts and field notes were coded and categorised by attaching one/more keywords representing the various themes (Spradley 1979), i.e. parents' perceptions of the internet, parents' religious beliefs, parents' internet use and parental mediation styles. Interpreting the data included 'critical thinking' beyond a structuring of the manifest meanings and connecting the meaning to cultural contexts and theoretical frameworks (Kvale and Brinkmann 2009).

Mothers' Perceptions of the Internet

Our informants were most concerned about three categories of internet risks: 'content', 'contact' and 'conduct' risk (Ponte and Simões 2009). On 'content risk', as observed by Stout (2001), our informants were deeply troubled by the apparent immorality of the internet, with the easy availability of online pornography being the greatest cause for concern. Without exception, all our informants believe that online pornography can cause moral degradation, spiritual corruption and self-destruction, as exemplified by this quote:

> I do not want my child to access pornographic sites. That what I'm concerned about since pornography is easily accessed. That's what I avoid most, worry about most. Using certain search terms like 'Barbie', pornographic pictures might appear. If children are not careful, they can accidentally access pornography. I am afraid pornography will damage their moral values. (Respondent 19, 41, undergraduate, housewife, 3 children, member of *Aisyiyah*)

Besides pornography, our informants (most of whom don the *jilbab*, a head covering which reveals only their face) also expressed grave reservations about the profusion of online images of immodestly dressed people revealing *aurat* (intimate parts of the body). Moreover, they worried that such content would undermine their children's faith:

> I always advise my child that posting a photograph of yourself in stylish and sexy dress is the same as selling oneself. (Respondent 14, 48, undergraduate, producer of Islamic magazine, 4 children, member of Aisyiah)

Some mothers were also discomfited by the fact that their children's exposure to online content had apparently led them to question Islamic beliefs. They found such situations troubling because they felt inadequate about their ability to address such doubts:

> My child likes to ask about Islamic dress. She asked me why we have to wear *hijab* (headdress). She saw on the internet many pictures of women with no *hijab*. So she asked me, 'What is the *hijab* for?' She also wondered about someone in the Middle East whose hand was chopped off for committing theft. She read the news on the internet. She asked, 'why must the hand be cut? Will Indonesian Muslims' hands be cut too if they steal?' Well, I said that every country is different. Sometimes I find it hard to explain [such matters] and have to ask my husband to help. (Respondent 49, 36, graduate, teacher, 2 children, activist of family-welfare education)

On 'contact risk', our informants expressed discomfort about the internet facilitating *haram* (forbidden) behaviour such as close and intimate conversations between unmarried couples via online platforms:

> I remind them [my children] that chatting online is mostly abused for ulterior motives [to seduce someone] and approximates adultery…which is forbidden for Muslims. (Respondent 11, 35, undergraduate, housewife, 2 children, member of an Islamic gathering)

As for 'conduct risk', most informants perceived that the internet promotes other negative qualities and behaviour in children including addictiveness, laziness, narcissism and aggression. Some informants also felt that the internet had an adverse activity displacement effect because their children prefer to stay at home to surf the internet rather than go outside with their friends, therefore lacking socialisation opportunities. A minority also found their children too heavily dependent on the internet for information and with an unhealthy predisposition for instant gratification:

> They can search for what they want by just clicking. Although the internet has a good side, in my opinion, children tend to struggle because of it. They are not interested in reading a book. They want to get everything quickly, practically, instantly. (Respondent 15, 36, junior college, 2 children)

In spite of these negative perceptions, our informants perceived the internet to be a valuable fount of knowledge and a veritable force for upward mobility. They believed that the internet will only assume greater importance in the future and that they need to equip their children with the necessary skills and competence to avail of this technology.

> For my husband and me, having internet access at home and permitting the child to use the internet is a kind of education. The future is the digital era. If our children are not introduced to the internet, they might be left behind. What a pity! The proof: after they knew

about YouTube, they got a lot of creative ideas and posted them in YouTube too. (Respondent 16, 34, graduate, police, 2 children)

Indeed, some informants shared that they had introduced the internet to their children from an early age. Most of them also utilised the internet to support parental obligations such as helping their children with their school projects. They also used the internet to satisfy their own curiosity about different issues and acknowledged that the internet had increased their religious knowledge and made them more conscious of the greatness of *Allah* (God):

> I am often amazed with the universe, the natural phenomena which are explained on internet. I started to understand, from the perspective of science, what is happening [in the universe]. From the perspective of religion, I acknowledge the magnificence of The Very Creator, more than before. (Respondent 26, 40, junior college, entrepreneur, 2 children)

Some informants also stated that *dakwah* (preaching) on the internet was more interesting than that on television, finding the internet advantageous because they could exercise greater control over its content:

> I prefer internet over TV because there are many bad things on TV. TV is more commercial and less educational. With the internet, [the benefits derived] depend on what users access and how they use this technology. (Respondent 5, 39, junior college, teacher, 4 children, member of *Aisyiah*)

Parental Mediation Strategies

Hence, the mothers were clearly cognizant of the internet's concurrent risks and opportunities and, despite the possible pitfalls, wanted their children to acquire what they considered to be important technological competencies. However, these mothers' desires were not matched by their own technical skills. To begin with, only a few mothers in our sample were frequent internet users, with many preferring to use other media such as television or print. Some of them explained that they rarely access the internet because of their limited knowledge and rudimentary online skills. The burdens of running the household and minding their children also did not leave them much time for the internet. On the occasions that they went online, it was to seek information and entertainment, communicate with friends and family, perform work-related tasks or just to pass the time. With comparatively limited exposure to the internet, many of our informants felt that they were *gaptek* (technology illiterate) and did not wish the same upon their children:

> It is now the internet era. Prohibiting children from accessing the internet will make them resemble their mother who does not know anything (chuckles). I admit that I am *gaptek* (technology illiterate), so I don't want my children become like me. All we need is to implant in them the values of religion so that they do not fall for technology. Technology is utilized to make our work easier, to enhance our knowledge. We have to be able to control technology, not the reverse, or our morality will deteriorate. (Respondent 28, 43, undergraduate, teacher, 4 children, manager of *Muallimat* – an Islamic seminary)

To this end, our informants sought to mediate their children's internet use so that the children could be well exposed to the medium but protected from its perceived ills. Most of them did not apply just a single strategy but a combination of restrictive, co-use, and active mediation strategies. Some would draw on religious authority in reminding their children of the Islamic value system of *pahala* (reward) and *dosa* (sin) when their children surfed the internet. Mothers who were more inclined towards restrictive mediation tended to hold strong assumptions about the internet being responsible for their children's bad behaviour. These mothers imposed strict rules limiting internet access to no more than 2 hours a day, except on weekends, holidays or when using the internet to complete school projects. They also prohibited internet use between 6 and 7 pm, the official prayer time for West Indonesia, during which they would ask their children to pray and study the *Qur'an*. They would also restrict access to particular types of content, with pornographic content being uniformly restricted across our informant pool. They also punished their children if they disobeyed, by forcibly turning off internet access or by withholding their allowances.

Apart from temporal and content restrictions, many informants also confined household internet access to specific locations within the home. The preferred location for computers with internet connections was the living room as it is a shared communal space. Some parents also placed the computer in a shared study or in their own bedrooms so that the children could only access the internet when the parents were at home. Most informants also forbade their children from going to internet cafés unsupervised because they see cafés as venues which promote vices such as smoking and pornography and where the *haram* (forbidden) activity of courtship may take place. In fact, it was the unsavoury nature of internet cafés that prompted some of our informants to install home internet access in the first place. Some informants preferred co-use strategies such as checking on the content of websites that their children accessed to ensure that the content was 'safe'. Others watched over their children when they surfed the internet. Some fathers, given their stronger technical prowess, would also periodically check the browsing history to know what their children did online.

On the other hand, a minority of informants were fairly relaxed about their children's internet use, vesting in their children autonomy and personal responsibility. These mothers argued that they did not need to impose strict rules because their children were cognizant of the types of online content they should refrain from accessing. They also felt that strict rules would in fact be counterproductive and alienating, adversely affecting their relationship with their children:

> I'm not too strict about the rules, just flexible. They already know what to do with the internet and understand the difference between appropriate and inappropriate content. Sometimes I just give them advice. I also compromise if they want they spend more time online. I'm worried my children will stay away from me if I'm too strict to them. (Respondent 44, 45, undergraduate, teacher, 2 children, *Qur'an* study).

Balancing Religious Ideals with Practical Realities

The contradictions that our informants experienced in their apprehensions about the internet and their concurrent appreciation for its benefits are not peculiar to Muslims. Parents of all nationalities, races and creeds have expressed concerns about the internet's negative dimensions, while profiting from its advantages (Vestby 1996; Livingstone and Bober 2006; Livingstone 2007a, b; Lim 2008). However, what is particularly challenging for the Indonesian Muslim mothers in our sample is the pressure on them to reconcile the growing pervasiveness of the internet with the pious religious climate in which they live. Our informants' religious ideals were shaped not only by personal experience but also by the influence of religious elders such as *ustadz* or *ustadzah* (male or female preachers), media activists, academics, teachers, psychologists, husbands, friends and family.

As the aforementioned sections show, Islamic values shaped the mothers' perceptions of the internet and the mediation strategies which they imposed. Our informants subscribe to the Islamic belief that supervision and guidance of children is a parental obligation. Children are regarded as a gift of *Allah* (God) and have to be nurtured to obey and spread the word of God, a process which Muslims believe should begin in childhood:

> In the Qur'an, it is clearly stated that the parents' responsibility for educating their children should be continued even until the afterlife. To educate children, it can mean many things – not only by providing formal education but also about educating them about [religious] devotion, and directing them in their media use to nurture their morality. (Respondent 16, 34, graduate, policewoman, 2 children)

Indeed, some mothers used Islamic law as a guide for supervising their children's internet use:

> [Of course] the Qur'an and Hadith do not explicitly mention the internet, but generally they outline general constraints. Sometimes, the internet has a great deal of content that contradicts the tenets of Islam such as pornography. We have to refer to the Qur'an and Hadith to evaluate the content. (Respondent 19, 41, undergraduate, housewife, 3 children, member of *Aisyiyah*)

The rapid growth of 'secular' and international media in Indonesia, made more accessible by the internet, further challenge Indonesian Muslim parents' attempts to raise their children in accordance with Islamic beliefs. Going beyond restricting and supervising their children's media consumption, the more avowedly religious families in our study would place greater emphasis on the observance of Islamic rituals so as to strengthen the family's Muslim identity, apparently as a bulwark against the corrosiveness of non-Islamic media content. They would also enrol their children in Islamic schools so as to strengthen their religious foundations. As Clark (2004) observed, such identity assertion is an effort to instil a perceptible distance between personal beliefs and those of external sources such as the media.

Informants who were less intensely involved in religious activities knew how to be 'normatively religious' but were less influenced by Islamic beliefs in their internet use and mediation. They preferred to draw upon general ethical principles and social norms so as to provide their children with more rational explanations for why particular types of online content or online activity were prohibited. Such informants tended to employ more secular terms such as *tidak pantas* (inappropriate) and *tidak mendidik* (devoid of educational merit) when assessing the appropriateness of online content, unlike their more avowedly religious counterparts who used religious terminology such as *haram* (forbidden) and *dosa* (sin). Indeed, these informants did not resist non-Islamic media but saw it as an edifying complement to their media repertoire:

> We as Muslims need other more general media. It is because we are living in a diverse environment with people from different religions. We need to mingle with those who are different from us. We also need to take a gaze at other types of knowledge so that we can properly place ourselves in an environment inhabited not only by us, the Muslims, but also by others. For me, general media help us [Muslims] to understand others and it's also an instrument for introspection to be a good Muslim (Respondent 38, undergraduate, researcher, 2 children).

Secularisation theory argues that Muslims are traditional holders of religious values and tend to be sceptical about the media (Buddenbaum and Stout 1996). Yet, as Hall (1997) argues, amidst the dominant discourse in which new technology insinuates its way into human lives, there is always a space in which people negotiate the media. Even within the Islamic movement, there is a recognition that Muslims cannot continually resist the media because these communication channels mediate religion, help to spread religious messages and serve as a platform for expressing and asserting one's Muslim identity, while developing a public sphere for the advancement of Islamic issues (Fealy and White 2008).

Conclusion

Our research focused on an understudied population – Muslim mothers in Indonesia – to understand their experiences of mediating their children's internet use in a society that strongly subscribes to religious ideals, while embracing technological advancements. In so doing, we sought to explore and elucidate upon the challenges that these women face as they seek to control and employ the internet. To them, the internet is a powerful medium which can have deleterious effects on one's faith and morality but, if correctly used, can significantly improve the quality of life for their families. While moral panic about the internet and unhealthy online content have been witnessed in many countries, the religious polemic surrounding these issues has set broad moral and religious norms about how children's internet use should be governed. Muslim mothers are left holding the fort within the domestic realm of children's internet consumption and have had to devise different mediation strategies to ensure that their children use the internet in positive ways that are congruent with Islamic principles. Our findings have illustrated how these women's faith influences their perceptions of the internet, both positive and negative, and informed their mediation strategies. While more religious families have sought to strengthen their faith to meet the onslaught of un-Islamic internet and media content, less devout Muslims see alternative media as beneficial and horizon broadening, thereby welcoming rather than resisting them.

This study has several limitations. It was conducted in Yogyakarta-Indonesia (a semi-urban–rural area) in which society is characterised by strong kinship ties and religion plays an important role in guiding people in their daily lives. So it is not surprising that many Muslim mothers in this city still hold their religious beliefs as the main reference point for parental mediation. Future studies should extend to Muslim families staying in urban as well as rural areas so as to facilitate comparative analysis. Furthermore, the study sought only the opinions of mothers. The views of Indonesian children and their perceptions of the mediation strategies imposed by their parents would afford a more complete picture of the phenomenon.

References

Abanto, F. L. (2004). *Children's and parents' perception towards TV programs and the practice of parental mediation*. Retrieved from http://www.bu.ac.th/knowledgecenter/epaper/july_dec2004/abanto.pdf

Alters, D. F. (2004). At the heart of the culture: The Hartmans and the Roelofs. In S. M. Hoover, L. S. Clark, & D. F. Alters (Eds.), *Media, home, and family* (pp. 103–129). New York: Routledge.

Anderson, M., & Shrum, W. (2007). Circumvention and social change: ICTs and the discourse of empowerment. *Women's Studies in Communication, 30*(2), 229–253.

Armfield, G. G., & Holbert, R. L. (2003). The relationship between religiosity and Internet use. *Journal of Media and Religion, 2*(3), 129–144.

Austin, E. W. (1993). Exploring the effects of active parental mediation of television content. *Journal of Broadcasting & Electronic Media, 37*(2), 146–158.

Austin, E. W., Roberts, D. F., & Nass, C. I. (1990). Influences of family communication on children's television-interpretation processes. *Communication Research, 17*(4), 545–564.

Bakardjieva, M., & Smith, R. (2001). The internet in everyday life computer networking from the standpoint of the domestic user. *New Media & Society, 3*(1), 67–83.

Bano, A. (2003). *Status of women in Islamic society* (Vol. 1). New Delhi: Anmol Publications.

BPS-Statistic of D.I. Yogyakarta Province. (2010). Daera Istimewa Yogyakarta Dalam Angka in Figures 2010. Retrieved from http://yogyakarta.bps.go.id/website/pdf_publikasi/Daerah-Istimewa-Yogyakarta-Dalam-Angka-2010.pdf

Buddenbaum, J. M., & Stout, D. A. (1996). Religion and mass media use: A review of the mass communication and sociology literature. In *Religion and mass media: Audiences and adaptations* (pp. 12–34).Thousand Oaks: Sage Publications.

Bull, B. W. (2005). The first full TV generation: A grounded theory study of persons born from 1960 to 1976 regarding their experiences with parental mediation of television and movies. Ph.D. Dissertation, University of Tennessee. http://trace.tennessee.edu/utk_graddiss/1870

Bybee, C. R., Robinson, D., & Turow, J. (1982). Determinants of parental guidance of children's television viewing for a special subgroup: Mass media scholars. *Journal of Broadcasting & Electronic Media, 26*(3), 697–710.

Clark, L. S. (2004). Being distinctive in a mediated environment: The Ahmeds and the Paytons. In *Media, home, and family* (pp. 79–102). New York: Routledge.

Croucher, S. M., Oommen, D., & Steele, E. L. (2009). An examination of media usage among French-Muslims. *Journal of Intercultural Communication Research, 38*(1), 41–57.

Croucher, S. M., Oommen, D., Borton, I., Anarbaeva, S., & Turner, J. S. (2010). The influence of religiosity and ethnic identification on media use among Muslims and non-Muslims in France and Britain. *Mass Communication and Society, 13*(3), 314–334.
Dholakia, R. R. (2006). Gender and IT in the household: Evolving patterns of Internet use in the United States. *The Information Society, 22*(4), 231–240.
Dorr, A., Kovaric, P., & Doubleday, C. (1989). Parent–child co-viewing of television. *Journal of Broadcasting & Electronic Media, 33*(1), 35–51.
Fadhal, S., Zarksasi, I., & Monik, S. (2011). Implementasi dan Tantangan Kegiatan Literasi Media Di Indonesia Sebagai Suatu Gerakan Sosial: Studi Perspektif Penggagas dan Target Kegiatan Literasi Media Di Jakarta dan Yogyakarta. In M. Nazaruddin & K. A. Saputro (Eds.), *Literasi Media Di Indonesia* (pp. 229–266). Yogyakarta: Komunikasi UII.
Fealy, G., & White, S. (Eds.). (2008). Introduction. In *Expressing Islam: Religious life and politics in Indonesia* (pp. 1–12). Singapore: Institute of Southeast Asian Studies (ISEAS) Publishing.
Flynn, B. (2003). Geography of the digital hearth. *Information Communication & Society, 6*(4), 551–576.
Frissen, V. A. (2000). ICTs in the rush hour of life. *The Information Society, 16*(1), 65–75.
Gentile, D. A., Saleem, M., & Anderson, C. A. (2007). Public policy and the effects of media violence on children. *Social Issues and Policy Review, 1*(1), 15–61.
Golan, G. J., & Day, A. G. (2010). In God we trust: Religiosity as a predictor of perceptions of media trust, factuality, and privacy invasion. *American Behavioural Scientist, 54*(2), 120–136.
Guntarto, B. (2011). Perkembangan Program Literasi Media Di Indonesia. In M. Nazaruddin & K. A. Saputro (Eds.), *Literasi Media Di Indonesia* (pp. 157–192). Yogyakarta: Komunikasi UII.
Hall, S. (1997). Introduction. In *Representation: Cultural representations and signifying practices* (pp. 1–12). London: Sage Publications.
Hamilton, N. F., & Rubin, A. M. (1992). The influence of religiosity on television viewing. *Journalism & Mass Communication Quarterly, 69*(3), 667–678.
Hidayat, D. (2003). Fundamentalisme Pasar dan Konstruksi Sosial Industri Penyiaran: Kerangka Teori Mengamati Pertarungan Di Sektor Penyiaran. In E. Gazali (Ed.), *Konstruksi Sosial Industri Penyiaran (Plus Acuan Tentang Penyiaran Publik & Komunitas)* (pp. 1–27). Jakarta: Departemen Ilmu Komunikasi Fisip UI.
Hynes, D., & Rommes, E. (2006). Fitting the Internet into our lives: IT courses for disadvantaged users. In *Domestication of media and technology* (pp. 125–144). Berkshire: Open University Press.
Ida, R. (2009). *Imaging Muslim women in Indonesian Ramadan soap operas*. Chiang Mai: Asian Muslim Action Network.
Indonesia-Investments. (n.d.-a). Religion in Indonesia. http://www.indonesia-investments.com/culture/religion/item69. Accessed 22 July 2015.
Indonesia-Investments. (n.d.-b). Unemployment in Indonesia. http://www.indonesia-investments.com/finance/macroeconomic-indicators/unemployment/item255. Accessed 22 July 2015.
Kazmi, F. (1994). Muslim socials and the female protagonist: Seeing a dominant discourse at work. In *Forging identities: Gender, communities, and the state* (pp. 226–243).New Delhi: Kali for Women.
Kitley, P. (2000). *Television, nation, and culture in Indonesia* (Vol. 104). Ohio: University Centre for International Studies.
Kulik, L. (2004). Predicting gender role ideology among husbands and wives in Israel: A comparative analysis. *Sex Roles, 51*(9–10), 575–587.
Kvale, S. (1996). *InterViews: An introduction to qualitative research interviewing*. Thousand Oaks: Sage Publications.
Kvale, S., & Brinkmann, S. (2009). *Interviews: Learning the craft of qualitative research interviewing*. Thousand Oaks: Sage Publications.

Lemor, A. R. (2006). Making a 'home'. The domestication of information and communication technologies in single parents' households. *Domestication of media and technology* (pp. 165–181). Maidenhead: Open University Press.

Lim, S. S. (2008). Technology domestication in the Asian homestead: Comparing the experiences of middle class families in China and South Korea. *East Asian Science, Technology and Society, 2*(2), 189–209.

Lin, C. A., & Atkin, D. J. (1989). Parental mediation and rulemaking for adolescent use of television and VCRs. *Journal of Broadcasting & Electronic Media, 33*(1), 53–67.

Livingstone, S. (2007a). Strategies of parental regulation in the media-rich home. *Computers in Human Behaviour, 23*(2), 920–941.

Livingstone, S. (2007b). *UK children go online: Balancing the opportunities against the risks*. Retrieved from http://eprints.lse.ac.uk/4035/

Livingstone, S., & Bober, M. (2006). Regulating the internet at home: Contrasting the perspectives of children and parents. In *Digital generations: Children, young people, and new media* (pp. 93–113). Mahwah: Lawrence Erlbaum Associates.

Livingstone, S., & Helsper, E. J. (2008). Parental mediation of children's internet use. *Journal of Broadcasting & Electronic Media, 52*(4), 581–599.

Messaris, P. (1982). Parents, children and television. In *Inter/media* (3rd ed., pp. 519–536). New York: Oxford University Press.

Mir-Hosseini, Z. (1998). Rethinking gender: Discussions with Ulama in Iran. *Critique: Journal for Critical Studies of the Middle East, 7*(13), 45–59.

Na, M. (2001). The home computer in Korea: Gender, technology, and the family. *Feminist Media Studies, 1*(3), 291–306.

Na, W., Son, Y., & Marshall, R. (1998). An empirical study of the purchase role structure in Korean families. *Psychology & Marketing, 15*(6), 563–576.

Nathanson, A. I. (2001). Parent and child perspectives on the presence and meaning of parental television mediation. *Journal of Broadcasting & Electronic Media, 45*(2), 201–220.

Notten, N., & Kraaykamp, G. (2009). Parents and the media: A study of social differentiation in parental media socialization. *Poetics, 37*(3), 185–200.

Nur, T. (2011). Pendidikan Kritis Media untuk Anak-Anak melalui Sinergitas Komunitas Pengajian dan Sekolah. In M. Nazaruddin & K. A. Saputro (Eds.), *Literasi Media Di Indonesia* (pp. 45–70). Yogyakarta: Komunikasi UII.

Oey-Gardiner, M. (2002). And the winner is… Indonesian women in public life. In K. Robinson & S. Bessel (Eds), *Women in Indonesia: Gender, equity and development* (pp. 100–112). Singapore: ISEAS Publishing.

On Device Research. (2013). Indonesia: The social media capital of the world. https://ondeviceresearch.com/blog/indonesia-social-media-capital-world. Accessed 22 July 2015.

Pasquier, D. (2001). Media at home: Domestic interactions and regulation. In S. Livingston & M. Bovrill (Eds), *Children and their changing media environment: A European comparative study* (pp. 161–179). Mahwah: Erlbaum Associates.

Peacock, J. L. (1978). *Purifying the faith: The Muhammadijah movement in Indonesian Islam*. Menlo Park: Benjamin-Cummings Publishing Company.

Ponte, C., & Simões, J. A. (2009). *Asking parents about children's internet use: Comparing findings about parental mediation in Portugal and other European countries*. EU kids online-final conference, London. Retrieved from http://www2.fcsh.unl.pt/eukidsonline/docs/Asking%20parents-FINAL%20Paper1_27-05-09.pdf

Rakow, L. F., & Navarro, V. (1993). Remote mothering and the parallel shift: Women meet the cellular telephone. *Critical Studies in Media Communication, 10*(2), 144–157.

Ribak, R. (2001). Like immigrants' negotiating power in the face of the home computer. *New Media & Society, 3*(2), 220–238.

Sarwono, B., Hendriyani & Guntarto, B. (2011). Efektivitas Pendidikan Media dalam Mengubah Konsumsi Media Anak: Eksperimen terhadap Siswa SD di Jawa Tengah dan Jawa Timur. In M. Nazaruddin & K. A. Saputro (Eds.), *Literasi Media Di Indonesia* (pp. 1–28). Yogyakarta: Komunikasi UII.

Sen, K., & Hill, D. T. (2007). *Media, culture and politics in Indonesia*. Singapore: Equinox Publishing.
Singh, S. (2001). Gender and the use of the Internet at home. *New Media & Society, 3*(4), 395–415.
Spradley, J. P. (1979). *The ethnographic interview*. New York: Holt, Rinehart and Winston
Stout, D. A. (2001). Beyond culture wars: An introduction to the study of religion and popular culture. In D. A. Stout & J. M. Buddenbaum (Eds.), *Religion and popular culture: Studies on the interaction of worldviews* (pp. 3–18). Ames: Iowa State University Press.
Stout, D. A., & Buddenbaum, J. M. (1996). Introduction: Towards a synthesis of mass communication research and the sociology of religion. In D. A. Stout & J. M. Buddenbaum (Eds.), *Religion and mass media: Audiences and adaptations* (pp. 3–11). Thousand Oaks: Sage Publications.
Stowasser, B. (1998). Gender issues and contemporary Quran interpretation. In Y. Y. Haddad & J. L. Esposito (Eds.), *Islam, gender, and social change* (pp. 30–44). New York: Oxford University Press.
Subiantoro, E. B. (2008). Perempuan Aceh Terus Mencari Keadilan. *Jurnal Perempuan, 57*, 21–31.
Sudarto. (2008). Peraturan Daerah dan Kearifan terhadap Perempuan. *Jurnal Perempuan, 57*, 7–18.
Sun, T. (2009). Parental mediation of children's TV viewing in China: An urban–rural comparison. *Young Consumers, 10*(3), 188–198.
Valkenburg, P. M., Krcmar, M., Peeters, A. L., & Marseille, N. M. (1999). Developing a scale to assess three styles of television mediation: "Instructive mediation," "restrictive mediation," and "social coviewing". *Journal of Broadcasting & Electronic Media, 43*(1), 52–66.
Van Doorn-Harder, N. (2002). The Indonesian Islamic debate on a woman president. *SOJOURN: Journal of Social Issues in Southeast Asia, 17*, 164–190.
Vestby, G. M. (1996). Technologies of autonomy? parenthood in contemporary 'modern times'. In M. Lie & K. H. Sorensen (Eds.), *Making technology our own* (pp. 65–90). Oslo: Scandinavian University Press.
Wanandi, J. (2002). Islam in Indonesia: Its history, development and future challenges. *Asia Pacific Review, 9*(2), 104–112.
Weaver, B., & Barbour, N. B. (1992). Mediation of children's televiewing. *Families in Society: The Journal of Contemporary Human Services, 73*(4), 236–242.

Chapter 4
Helping the Helpers: Understanding Family Storytelling by Domestic Helpers in Singapore

Kakit Cheong and Alex Mitchell

Abstract The recording and sharing of family stories remains an important aspect of what it means to be a "family". Existing research has shown that such stories help family members maintain close bonds. Additionally, the sharing of personal experiences can help family members create and present individual and family identities. Traditionally, these stories are shared face-to-face. However, for a variety of reasons, more families are geographically distributed. While there has been extensive research into how migrant workers make use of ICTs for social support or interpersonal communication, there remains a gap in understanding how these workers use ICTs specifically for family storytelling. To address this, we conducted two rounds of ethnographic interviews with 25 Filipino domestic helpers in Singapore. At the same time, we sought to examine the types of stories these women currently share. As such, we deployed cultural probe packs which consisted of a disposable camera and writing materials. The interview findings show that factors such as cost or limited access to technology resulted in fewer opportunities for family storytelling. In addition, interviewees also described themselves to have "nothing interesting to share" and that they were "unable to do more" in terms of sharing their experiences with their families back home. Interestingly, the cultural probe findings suggest that this perception may not always be accurate, as evidenced by how the participants were able to reflect upon their daily lives and record numerous personal experiences using the probes.

Keywords Mobile phones • Family storytelling • Domestic helpers • Migrant workers • Cultural probes

---

K. Cheong (✉) • A. Mitchell
National University of Singapore, Singapore
e-mail: c_kakit@hotmail.com; alexm@nus.edu.sg

Introduction

Family stories and storytelling remain an important part of what it means to be a "family". Apart from creating and maintaining close ties among family members (Bohanek et al. 2009; Taylor et al. 2013), family stories are necessary for individual and family identity formation (Fivush 2008; Fivush et al. 2010) and for sharing significant personal experiences that are intended to be remembered or retold (Dalsgaard et al. 2006; Pratt and Fiese 2004). Traditionally, such stories have been shared face-to-face during both formal and informal family gatherings (Stone 2004). However, in recent times, more families are geographically distributed, for example, migrant families where one or both parents work overseas for extended periods of time. Such families typically rely on information and communication technologies (ICTs) such as the mobile phone and computers to communicate. While there has been prior research examining how migrant workers make use of ICTs for social support or interpersonal communication, there remains a gap in understanding how such workers utilize ICTs for family storytelling. To address this, our study sought to understand whether and how domestic helpers in Singapore use ICTs to share family stories in their daily lives.

In Singapore, as with many other developed countries, more women are joining the workforce, resulting in the replacement of traditional structures where the husband was the sole breadwinner (Quek 2014). Recent statistics from the country's Ministry of Manpower (MOM) state that women currently comprise 58.1 % of the total labor force in Singapore (MOM 2014). Many of these families with two working parents employ female migrant workers, often referred to as domestic helpers or maids, to perform household duties such as cleaning the home, taking care of children or elderly family members, cooking, and grocery shopping. According to MOM, there are currently over 222,500 foreign domestic helpers from countries such as Indonesia, India, Myanmar, and the Philippines working in Singapore (MOM 2015). Unlike other migrant workers who work in the construction or manufacturing industries, these women are employed as "live-in" maids and are required to live with their employers. The nature of these women's working experience and hospitability of their work environment is largely determined by their employers and highly dependent on the quality of the employer-employee relationship. Not surprisingly, given these women's low socioeconomic status and the primarily menial nature of their work, there is a great power differential between them and their employers, with the latter being able to impose often onerous conditions on the former. For example, prior research suggests that maids are often restricted in terms of their access to technology (Thomas and Lim 2010) and are also discouraged by their employers from taking part in social activities outside of the house (Thomas and Lim 2010). In some cases, employers also utilise surveillance technologies like webcams to track their maids' movements and activities (Rahman et al. 2005). Given such restrictions, it is all the more important for these women to be able to communicate and share significant personal experiences with their families, considering how many of them are also mothers who have left behind their own children to work overseas (Madianou 2012).

In the rest of this paper, we first review the literature on the use of ICTs by migrant workers and prior research on family storytelling. Next, we describe our methodology, followed by a discussion of the findings, and we conclude by identifying areas for future research.

Literature Review

Prior literature relating to the present study can be broadly categorized into three groups: the use of ICTs by migrant workers, family storytelling and communication, and the use of ICTs for family storytelling.

Use of ICTs by Migrant Workers

There is a growing body of research focusing on the use of ICTs by migrant workers and their left-behind families. There are two dominant threads: ICT usage for mediated parenting and ICT usage for social support and interpersonal communication.

Studies in the first group show that more migrant workers, in particular, female migrant workers, are adopting the use of mobile phones to reconstruct their roles as parents by fulfilling motherly duties such as checking that their children have completed their homework or whether they are performing well in school (Cabanes and Acedera 2012; Madianou 2012; Madianou and Miller 2011). Other studies have explored how migrant workers use ICTs for social support (Alampay et al. 2013; Chib et al. 2013; Rahman et al. 2005), as well as for interpersonal communication (Thomas and Lim 2010; Thompson 2009). These studies argue that migrant workers maintain their mental health and psychological well-being to some extent with the help of ICTs. At the same time, it is important to note that ICTs may also affect migrant workers negatively (Thomas and Lim 2010). For example, due to cost, most domestic helpers choose to send text messages instead of calling. In addition, the families of such workers typically choose not to call their mothers and instead rely on "missed calling" to notify their parents that they need to speak. Such asymmetries in communication can lead to misunderstandings or frustrations (Madianou and Miller 2011). Furthermore, while mobile communications have allowed for perpetual contact, such technologies also result in "a state of perpetual concern for their children's well-being" (Lim and Soon 2010, p. 212).

Family Storytelling

Broadly speaking, a family story can be defined as "narrative accounts of personal experiences that have meaning to individuals and to the family as a whole" (Pratt and Fiese 2004, p. 1). As Kellas (2010) asserts, "family stories and storytelling are central to creating, maintaining, understanding and communicating personal relationships" (p. 1). For this paper, relevant literature about family stories can be categorized into two groups: sensemaking and identity formation.

The first group of research investigates how family stories and storytelling helps families to make sense of everyday events (Bohanek et al. 2009; Kellas 2010), as well as difficult or traumatic experiences (Kiser et al. 2010; Koenig Kellas and Trees 2006; Trees and Kellas 2009). For example, Kellas and Trees (2006) argue that through the process of telling a story together, family members are able to reach a "shared conclusion concerning the meaning of the experience" (p. 49). In other words, by sharing such stories, family members are able to discuss and shape the meaning of events (Roberts 1994). At the same time, such stories enable individual family members to make sense of their family relationships (Trees and Kellas 2009). Research in health psychology has also revealed that the act of sharing traumatic experiences positively affects an individual's well-being. As Pennebaker et al. (1988) put forward, the failure to confront traumatic experiences can lead to an individual experiencing greater levels of stress, which in turn may increase the incidence of illness. The same study also revealed that individuals showed improvements in physical health after they disclosed their traumatic experiences through writing (Pennebaker et al. 1988).

The second group of studies suggest that family stories are useful for constructing individual (Fivush 2007, 2008; Fivush et al. 2008, 2010) and family identity (Frensch et al. 2007; McCarthy 2012). Studies in this group have revealed different ways in which parents reminisce about daily events or experiences with their children and how such differences may be critical for a child's emotional understanding and well-being. For example, mothers who reminisce in more elaborative ways and encourage participation from other family members have children who show higher levels of emotional understanding and regulation (Fivush 2007; Fivush et al. 2006). While family stories and their messages affect young children in particular, research also shows that identity stories continue to develop and influence a person throughout his or her life (McAdams 2004). Identity stories have also been found to be positively associated with individual's ratings of subjective mental health, life satisfaction (Ackerman et al. 2000), and pro-social personality characteristics (Peterson and Klohnen 1995).

Use of ICTs in Family Storytelling

Finally, the third group of work explores how ICTs can be used specifically for family storytelling. Studies within this group typically explore how parents and children who are physically apart make use of ICTS to share personal stories (Wong-Villacres and Bardzell 2011; Wyche and Grinter 2012). In addition, other researchers have investigated how stories are recorded and shared between grandparents and grandchildren (Forghani and Neustaedter 2014; Vutborg et al. 2010). These studies reveal that family members, in particular the left-behind children, express a strong desire for in-depth interactions with their parents largely due to the fact they are not able to have shared experiences.

While there has been extensive research in all three areas, there remains a lacuna that can be valuably filled by the present study. Previous studies have focused on families whose members are physically proximate and of relatively high socioeconomic status, with ready access to ICTs. However, to the best of our knowledge, there has been no prior research investigating the use of ICTs in family storytelling by families who may not enjoy these privileges. To address this gap, our research focuses on low-waged Filipino migrant workers who are working in Singapore as domestic helpers, leaving their families behind in the Philippines. Our research was guided by the following questions:

1. Do domestic helpers use ICTs to record and share family stories, and if so, how?
2. What types of family stories are shared by such women?

Methodology

We conducted two rounds of semi-structured ethnographic interviews with 25 Filipino domestic helpers in Singapore. At the same time, we also deployed cultural probes to identify the types of stories domestic helpers currently share or would like to share. All participants were recruited through snowball sampling, which is useful for reaching difficult-to-locate subjects such as undocumented immigrants or migrant workers (Babbie 2013). In addition, given the sensitive nature of some stories, it was important for the researchers to build rapport with the interviewees before they would agree to participate in the study. All interviewees were recruited at two Catholic churches where these women congregate on Sundays.

In the first round of interviews, we explained our research goals to the interviewees and requested details on their age, family background, city of origin, and years spent working as a domestic helper in Singapore. We then asked them to describe which ICTs they used to communicate with their families. Special focus was given to whom in their family they spoke to most often and the types of stories they chose to share. Taking into consideration their unique work environments, we also asked them whether there were any stories or experiences that they wanted to share with their families, but were either unwilling or unable to do so.

After the interview, participants were provided with a cultural probe pack. According to Gaver et al. (1999), cultural probes are designed to "provoke inspirational responses" from participants (p. 21). He further explains that such probes provide "fragmentary clues about their lives and thoughts" and are "valuable in inspiring design ideas that could enrich people's lives in new and pleasurable ways" (Gaver et al. 2004, p. 53). As such, many researchers have utilized probes to reveal and gather tacit information in an unobtrusive way (Crabtree et al. 2003; Graham and Rouncefield 2008; Horst et al. 2004; Hutchinson et al. 2003). At the same time, we acknowledge the potential limitations of cultural probes. As McDougall and Fels (2010) argue, researchers have to be careful not to design probes that may contain biases. Other scholars have also pointed out that the researcher's absence while the probe is being deployed may mean that they are unable to ask participants questions while the probe is in use (Luusua et al. 2015). To avoid these pitfalls, we were careful not to create the probes based on any specific expectations. Instead, we designed our probe pack to enable participants to reflect on and record the different types of personal experiences or stories in their daily lives that they hoped to share with their families. Each probe pack consisted of a disposable camera that could capture up to 39 shots and writing materials (see Fig. 4.1). We gave participants suggestions for the use of the camera, such as capturing significant or new experiences, people, or places in their lives. We stressed that such suggestions were for inspiration only and that participants could be as creative as they liked in the usage of the items. In addition, we encouraged them to write down the specific story that each photo was supposed to tell. Participants were given about three weeks to make use of the probes.

Following this, we collected the probes back and developed the photos. The photos and stories were then used in the second round of interviews to prompt further discussion and allow us to delve deeper into the specific types of stories that participants wished to tell to their families.

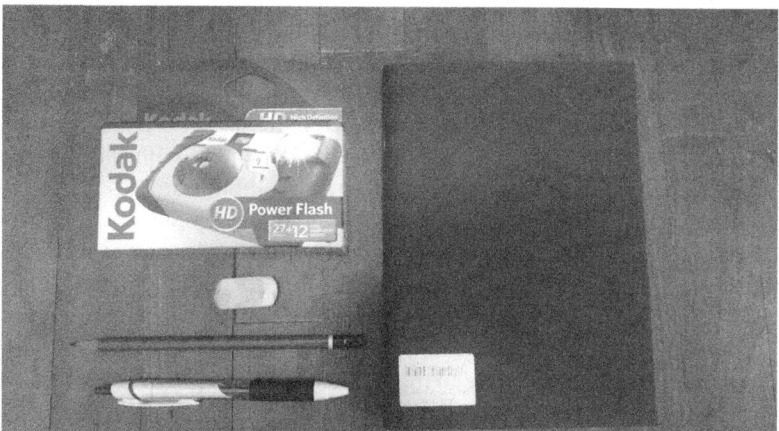

Fig. 4.1 Probe pack materials

Throughout the study, ethical guidelines were strictly followed. This included informing participants that they could withdraw from the study at any time, that their privacy and confidentiality would be respected, and that the interviews would only be audio recorded with their consent. The interviews were conducted in English in a location specified by the interviewee. The recordings were transcribed and analyzed using inductive coding. As (Seidman 2013) points out, inductive coding is useful for condensing raw textual data into a brief summary format and to establish clear links between research objectives and the summary findings from the raw data. For this chapter, we focus on the themes that emerged with regard to the domestic helpers' use of different ICTs for family storytelling.

Findings

Domestic Helpers Use of ICTs for Family Storytelling

The majority of our interviewees utilize a variety of technologies to share family stories, including the mobile phone, landline (albeit to a small extent), computers, and the Internet. While there were some variations in the frequency of use for each medium, most interviewees agreed that the mobile phone was the primary communicative device. They also shared that during their conversations with their families, they prioritized hearing updates from their families over sharing their own personal experiences. More importantly, we found that the types of technologies used for family storytelling by domestic helpers were largely determined by three factors: what technologies their employers permitted, what technologies their family back home had access to, and cost.

Our interviewees shared that their employers often dictated the types of technologies they were allowed to use, even if they were willing to purchase such devices on their own:

> During my first 1.5 years, my employer instructed the agency to include a clause in my contract that did not allow me to have a handphone or any 'off-days' [rest days] for two years, saying it will affect my work. One night, I cried and plead with them to let me call back as it is my daughter's birthday. I explain to them that they are parents also and that I am working for my daughter, so please let me call to wish her happy birthday. After that incident, my employers asked me to buy a mobile phone for myself. (Participant 8)

In most cases, the interviewees explained that they are often not permitted to use their mobile phones during "work hours," which typically last from 5am to 10pm. As a result, they shared that they are often exhausted and find it difficult to recount personal experiences to their families on weekdays.

More notably, it appears that for some employers, the "visibility" of the communicative device matters. Participant 3 shared that although she was permitted by her employer to use the household Wi-Fi for her mobile phone, when she wanted to use a tablet, her employers objected even though she intended to use the same applications and services: "Sir ok, but Ma'am not ok. She don't like me using big tablet." According to the interviewee, there was no reason given for this reservation, suggesting that some employers may be imposing restrictions based on their whims.

As a result of these limitations, our interviewees often choose to use their devices discreetly, even when prior permission had been given. On the other hand, a few participants also shared that they have learnt to use new forms of communication from members of their employer's family. As Participant 5 opined, "my employer daughter is the one who gave me Wi-Fi password and help me create FB (Facebook) account." Through this social media account, she is able to post photos of her life in Singapore, as well as share personal experiences with her parents. In other cases, some employers allow their helpers to use the household computer or mobile tablet on their days off. Even so, as Participant 1 shared, "I use but not so much because I don't want them to think I'm greedy."

The above quote suggests that given the power relations between employers and helpers, the latter may choose to use technologies that employers have provided only sparingly, for fear of judgment or criticism. At the same time, the same employers may not be comfortable with the helpers purchasing their own tablets, revealing their desire to restrict the helper's ICT usage. Participants also said that employers, in particular the female head of the household, would occasionally ask their helpers about the nature of their personal conversations. Hence, participants were careful not to openly share negative experiences with their left-behind family. This was so they could avoid having to lie about their phone conversations to their employers.

Our interviewees also shared that apart from the limitations set by their employers, the types of technology their own family had access to also influenced the types of ICTs they used for family storytelling. In one case, a participant (10) said that it was difficult just to call or text back as her parents resided in a mountainous region with poor cell phone reception. Most respondents also explained that due to the high cost of a monthly broadband plan, their families relied on prepaid top-up cards. Alternatively, some families still relied on using text messages to set up a time when the family member would travel to an internet café to talk.

We also found that at times, even if the family had access to a prepaid data card, some family members, in particular elderly parents, may not possess the technical knowledge to use certain technologies. In such cases, our participants rely on other members of the family to retell the stories or scaffold the sharing of experiences. For example, one shared how her mother did not know how to use Facebook and could only view photos when her other daughter came to visit. On her part, the participant (12) would send text messages to her sister with instructions on which photos to show her mother. At times, participants also expressed that they chose to limit the types of technologies that their children had access to. For example, some felt that their children were too young to have social media accounts or mobile phones, for fear that such technologies may serve as distractions from their studies. In other cases, mothers did not want to give their children mobile phones or tablets in case they became targets of crime. Madaniou and Miller (2011) coined the term "polymedia" to explain this need for "each relationship to create a configuration of usage generally employing several different media" (p. 125). However, as they explain, a state of polymedia is only achieved if three conditions are met: the individual has ready access to a wide range of at least half a dozen communication media, media literacy or the ability and knowledge to create content, and when the expense is mostly shifted to existing infrastructure, as opposed to a particular act of communication. Based on these criteria, very few of our participants appear to be at a stage that can be considered to be polymedia.

Finally, cost remains a barrier for helpers to share family stories with their loved ones:

> Sometimes when you talk on the phone, you cannot explain very well. In the mobile phone, very expensive, so you need to save money. (Participant 9)

Interestingly, to overcome this barrier, these women often make use of traditional means of recording their daily events and experiences, such as scrapbooks or diaries. With the exception of Participant 6, all of the interviewees shared that they kept a journal which they wrote regularly:

> My daily writings are about what makes me happy, what makes me sad, what encourages me, and writing to my future self, like my plans to go to Canada and study one day. (Participant 1)

While most interviewees acknowledge that such diaries were for themselves, many said that they intended to draw upon these entries to share personal experiences with their families upon returning home, suggesting that noncomputer-mediated forms of recording stories remain important, especially for such transnational families.

Stories for Sensemaking

Kellas (2010) opines that family storytelling is useful for sensemaking and navigating difficult experiences. We found that our interviewees used stories to explain why they needed to work overseas. Such stories were often targeted not only at their children but also at their husbands or parents who would try to persuade them to return home. In such circumstances, they would choose to repeat a particular story to reassure the other party:

> I am working to provide for you and your future, because your father cannot afford, don't have stable job, that's why I need to work. (Participant 2)

> I don't share with my father because I left to work without his approval, but I tell my mother that I work here for them and so I can take care of them. I tell her to remind him that I will come back when I save enough. (Participant 8)

Depending on whom the story was being shared with, it was common for interviewees to reassure the family member by painting a picture of future possibilities, outlining what they could do with the money they were earning overseas, so as to justify their collective sacrifice. For example, promises would be made to children of buying them toys or technological devices, such as mobile phones or laptops. In other cases, the story may include plans to rebuild their existing house or to buy a new house to "secure a future" (Participant 2).

Stories were also used by the participants to help their family members make sense of difficult experiences. For example, one interviewee said:

> My son call me and say 'cause he eat with whole family so not enough to eat, very hungry. I explain to him that when I work here, I also eat very little, but through God we can overcome this and I am working hard so when I come back can take care of you. (Participant 2)

Interestingly, the participant chose to withhold certain details about the story. For her, the story was intended to teach her son about the importance of sharing. However, when she spoke with her husband, she would be more open:

> I tell my husband that I cook for the whole family every day, but sometimes they eat finish all [the food], then I left with very little, so I also feel very sad. (Participant 2)

The above example suggests that the stories shared are adapted to different audiences. They would choose to reinforce their parental role by using their personal experiences as life lessons for their children or seek solace and support from their siblings, parents, or spouses.

Stories for Identity Formation

Apart from using stories for sensemaking, our interviewees also told and retold stories to construct specific identities, for example, as a religious, loving mother. All of the participants who had children insisted that it was important for their children to remember them as a "good Christian." As a result, many of the photos they captured with the probes revolved around their Sunday activities at church:

> It surprises me to know that not everyone is a child of god... It is very important that you know to whose family you belong [to]. The first step in becoming a member of god's family is an understanding of who God is and what he has done. (Participant 3)

> This bible was gift from my employer. I'm so blessed to having this book because I learned a lot from them. Through reading, sharing and encouraging of my employer and church mates, I become one of them. (Participant 5)

Arguably, such stories support Fivush's (2010) position that family stories are critical for the construction and reinforcement of individual and family identities. Given our recruitment method, our interviewees were active practitioners of their Catholic faith and would combine their personal experiences with religious teachings to portray themselves as appropriate role models for their children.

Types of Experiences Not Shared

While our primary focus was to investigate the types of family stories shared by helpers, we felt that it was also critical to delve into stories that the helpers were unable or unwilling to share and the underlying reasons for their omission. Interestingly, we found that they deliberately excluded numerous types of experiences from their usual conversations:

> I don't want to share with my children my troubles, it will affect the children. Also, husband care but so far apart, will only make him more worried. (Participant 4)

> Already they have a lot to think, I try not to, I don't want them to worry but of course simple things like I not feeling well, they cannot do anything, just pray for me. (Participant 6)

Other types of stories that were withheld by these women included reprimands from their employers, feminine health problems, and their love interests (for single women). For one interviewee, even positive experiences such as outings were kept from her children:

> 'cause if I told them (her children) I am going out with my friends, they feel like jealous and ask "why me cannot go out with my friends." (Participant 4)

While most participants, especially the mothers felt this way, other participants (2, 8) felt otherwise and shared that it was important to share "both the good and bad things" with their families in order to gain moral support. Given the sensitive nature of these stories, interviewees responded that these types of stories were usually shared with only one or two family members. Notably, it was common for them to share sensitive stories with their siblings. They felt that they could speak freely with their siblings about their problems without fear of causing additional worry for their family. It is also important to note that while our interviewees were not willing to share particular stories with their families while overseas, they expressed a strong desire to share these stories in the future. Based on the interviews, there appears to be two reasons for this desire for future family storytelling. Firstly, most of our interviewees expressed that they would only be able to engage in "true sharing" upon their return. For these women, face-to-face communication was still the best way to share about their lives. Next, some interviewees, in particular helpers who were mothers, explained that they were not currently able or willing to share particular stories with their children, as the latter were still too young to fully grasp the meaning of their stories.

Discovering Stories Not Previously Shared

During the first interview session, we noticed that the participants often claimed that they did not have many stories to share with their families, despite their strong desire to do so. To better understand this issue, we provided all participants with the probe packs to observe if there were events or experiences in their daily lives that could be recorded to be shared as a family story.

With the exception of one participant whose camera malfunctioned, all the other participants were highly motivated to complete the activity. Every helper took a minimum of ten photos, with many using the entire reel of 39 photos. These photos were then discussed during the follow-up interview session.

In general, most of the photos reflected the stories already identified earlier, such as their Sunday church activities, their daily chores, the occasional outing, the dishes they cooked, and so on (see Fig. 4.2). More interestingly, we found that some photos involved experiences or stories that had not previously been shared in any of their conversations.

As one participant wrote:

> This place is in my past two years, I'm always here at this place [see Figure 4.3] in Bedok Clearwater. After church I come here and read my daily bread and some textbook. I love this place, so quiet and fresh air. At this place I'm thinking of my children and then I talk to God. I cried because I miss my family. One time it [crying] happened here...while I'm walking, the ... man [a construction worker] following me and trying to take my number and I scold him. (Participant 7)

This excerpt reveals this participant's moments of quiet solitude when she enjoys a reprieve from her work to be one with her family, even if only in spirit. Notably, she had also protected her family from her negative experience of harassment, choosing not to mention it to them.

Describing a photo of the view from her bedroom window (see Fig. 4.4), another participant wrote:

> I choose to take this photo because this place makes me confident if I am lonely or feel bored. I go stand by the window of my room so I can see all of these buildings, so I can think and see far from my employer house and become fresh my mind. It makes to gone my feeling lonely or boring. If I go back to my parent's house, I don't have a place like this. (Participant 10)

This account captures the introspective moments in this participant's working life, moments from which she draws stimulation and rejuvenation. By looking out of her bedroom window, she is virtually liberated from the physical boundaries of

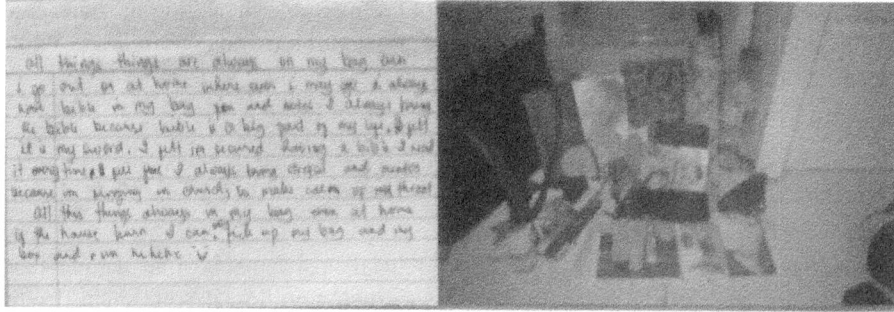

Fig. 4.2 Example of story and photo capture by participant using the probe pack

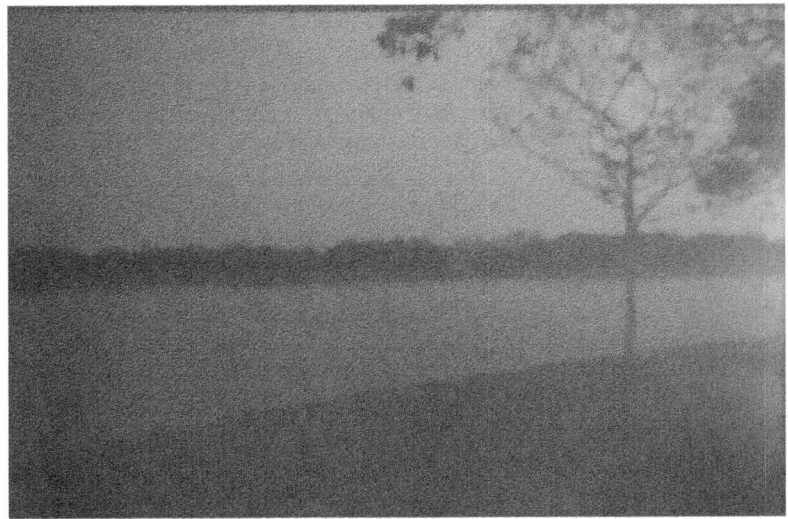

Fig. 4.3 Participant's photo of the park she frequented

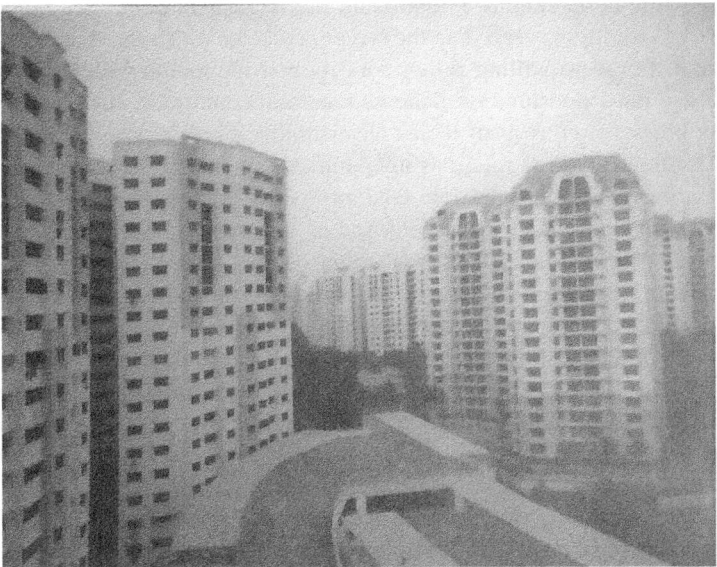

Fig. 4.4 Participant's photo from her bedroom window

her employer's home, thereby easing her feelings of loneliness and tedium. Again this is a personal story that she keeps to herself and does not share with loved ones, perhaps because it reflects the greyer aspects of her working life that she does not wish to burden them with.

After the probes, the interviewees mused that even though their mobile phones had built-in cameras which they often used, the probe spurred them to reflect upon their daily activities and experiences in different and unprecedented ways, enabling them to compare how their lives had changed both positively and negatively. Furthermore, all the participants expressed that they intended to continue reflecting on their daily experiences to share new stories with their families. As Participant 10 said, "these photos and stories let me show my children and family what Singapore is like, which they may never see."

Discussion

To better understand the implications of our study, we will attempt to situate our findings within the broader landscape of existing literature. First, by uncovering if and how domestic helpers use ICTs to record and share family stories, our study adopts a different lens to examine ICT use by migrant workers. We identified three determinants of the types of ICTs used: what employers permit, what technologies migrant workers' families can access, and cost considerations. Interestingly, we noted that while cost remains a significant barrier, our interviewees reported that their working conditions served as the larger obstacle. We found that even in cases where employers were willing to temporarily provide maids with communicative devices, these rare opportunities came with certain conditions, such as letting their employers know the content of their conversations. Furthermore, given the power dynamics of their working relationships, domestic helpers often chose to use such devices sparingly. They also have to take into consideration the level of access that their family members back home enjoy. For example, some participants would rather not give their young children access to some devices, for fear of affecting their studies. In such cases, they chose to forgo opportunities for better communication and developed strategies to overcome their limited ICT access, resonating with findings from previous studies such as those of Yeoh and Huang (1998).

Secondly, our study also contributes to the literature on family storytelling as we found that traditional, noncomputer-mediated technologies still play an important role in the lives of the women we studied. Most of our interviewees chose to record their daily experiences on traditional journals or scrapbooks, with the aim of sharing these stories in the future. In the same vein, other studies on family storytelling by migrant workers have noted that transnational families adopt creative adaptations to circumvent technological constraints (Wyche and Grinter 2012). In some cases, interviewees also noted that some experiences, in particular negative ones, were not suitable for sharing with their young children. However, they pledged to share such stories during opportune moments as they hope such stories about themselves will be remembered. We also find strong evidence that our interviewees share particular personal experiences for the purposes of sensemaking and maintaining specific identities with their significant others. This is supported by how they would often tailor the content of each story to suit the intended audience. Again, these women are often ready to put their own needs and wishes aside, choosing not to share negative experiences to avoid worrying their family members.

Finally, the probes also uncovered noteworthy findings. During the interviews, participants often claimed that they did not have many interesting personal experiences to share and that they were "unable to do more." However, their eagerness to tell stories using the probe photos suggests that they actually *do* have stories to share, but simply do not realize that they do. One possible explanation for this incongruence could be the looking glass theory which postulates that an individual's "self" grows out of his or her social interactions with others. In other words, individuals are likely to shape their self-concepts based on how others perceive them (Cooley 1902). Therefore, it is possible that given their limited opportunities for social interaction, domestic helpers feel that their lives of repetitive drudgery do not merit discussion. Prior research has shown that domestic helpers are a marginalized group in Singapore who are typically discouraged by employers from partaking in social activities outside of the house (Yeoh and Huang 1998). Arguably therefore, given their circumscribed experience and worldview, these women were not naturally inclined to viewing themselves as individuals with personal stories worth telling or repeating.

Methodologically, our experience showed that the probes were valuable for revealing insights beyond more traditional research methods. However, we faced several challenges which future researchers may wish to take into consideration. Firstly, as mentioned earlier, probes have to be carefully designed to ensure that they do not include assumptions or biases. As McDougall and Fels (2010) opine, probes that are built on researchers' biases are likely to be ineffective, since researchers will learn nothing beyond what they already assumed. In our study, the probes were carefully redesigned several times to eliminate preconceptions or expectations. For example, even though we were interested in family storytelling, we did not specify any particular interpretation of what constitutes a "family story." Secondly, the analysis of data from probes can prove challenging as researchers may not always understand the full meaning of a particular text. To avert this situation, we used the second round of interviews to ask the participants follow-up questions. Consequently, we did not encounter significant problems with the data coding and analysis.

Conclusion

This study sought to examine how domestic helpers make use of ICTs to create and share family stories. Our study revealed that given their constrained working environments and limited social interaction, our participants often felt that they are unable to share much about their lives. As such, these helpers sought to make the "best" use of their communication time to share specific types of family stories. These stories were intended to help family members make sense of their migrant work experience, as well as to construct and reinforce positive family identities. More importantly, our probe pack findings suggest that domestic helpers do have a variety of stories they wish to share with their families, despite initially believing the opposite about themselves. Our next step is to help the helpers by developing a family storytelling mobile application, in an effort to facilitate domestic helper's communication and relationship nurturance with their left-behind families (Cheong and Mitchell 2015). To do so, we will be deploying additional probes and conducting participatory sessions to design the application. We also intend to evaluate the strengths and weaknesses of the application through qualitative user studies.

This study has uncovered meaningful insights into how domestic helpers use ICTs to share family stories. However, future research may seek to explore the experiences of migrant workers in different vocations and working environments. Furthermore, we have only been able to investigate how family stories are shared from the perspective of mothers. It would be useful to approach the research topic from multiple perspectives to see how each family member experiences and retells specific family stories.

Acknowledgments This research is supported by the National Research Foundation, Prime Minister's Office, Singapore, under its International Research Centre @ Singapore Funding Initiative and administered by the Interactive & Digital Media Programme Office.

Appendix: Profile of Interviewees

Name	Age	Marital status	No. of children/age	Technologies used	Time spent overseas
Participant 1	24	Single	None	Mobile phone, email	3 months
Participant 2	34	Married	2 (12, 8)	Mobile phone, Facebook	5 years
Participant 3	34	Separated	1 (13)	Mobile phone, Facebook	1 year
Participant 4	39	Married	2 (10, 8)	Mobile phone, Skype, Facebook	9 years
Participant 5	37	Single	None	Mobile phone, Facebook	4 years
Participant 6	46	Single	None	Mobile phone	22 years
Participant 7	36	Married	3 (12, 11, 9)	Mobile phone, Facebook	3 years
Participant 8	28	Married	1 (8)	Mobile phone, Skype, Facebook	2 years
Participant 9	42	Married	3 (11, 10, 8)	Mobile phone, Facebook	3 years
Participant 10	30	Single	None	Mobile phone, email, Facebook	4 years
Participant 11	29	Married	1 (12)	Mobile phone, Facebook	2 years
Participant 12	30	Single	None	Mobile phone	6 years

(continued)

Name	Age	Marital status	No. of children/age	Technologies used	Time spent overseas
Participant 13	31	Married	2 (10, 2)	Mobile phone, Skype, WeChat	2 years
Participant 14	46	Married	None	Mobile phone	8 years
Participant 15	30	Single	None	Mobile phone	6 years
Participant 16	31	Mother	2 (11, 8)	Mobile phone, Facebook	2 years
Participant 17	38	Mother	2 (9, 11)	Mobile phone, Facebook, WeChat	4 years
Participant 18	32	Mother	1 (6)	Mobile phone	5 years
Participant 19	32	Mother	1 (12)	Mobile phone	2 years
Participant 20	28	Single	None	Mobile phone, Facebook	1 year
Participant 21	29	Single	None	Mobile phone, WeChat, Facebook	4 years
Participant 22	27	Single	None	Mobile phone, Facebook	2 years
Participant 23	31	Single	None	Mobile phone, Facebook	2 years
Participant 24	27	Single	None	Mobile phone, WeChat, Facebook	1 year
Participant 25	36	Mother	2 (16, 11)	Mobile phone, Facebook	7 years

References

Ackerman, S., Zuroff, D. C., & Moskowitz, D. (2000). Generativity in midlife and young adults: Links to agency, communion, and subjective well-being. *The International Journal of Aging and Human Development, 50*(1), 17–41.

Alampay, E., Alampay, L., & Raza, K. (2013). *The impact of cybercafés on the connectedness of children left behind by overseas Filipino workers*. Seattle: Technology & Social Change Group, University of Washington Information School.

Babbie, E. R. (2013). *The practice of social research*. Belmont: Wadsworth Cengage Learning.

Bohanek, J. G., Fivush, R., Zaman, W., Lepore, C. E., Merchant, S., & Duke, M. P. (2009). Narrative interaction in family dinnertime conversations. *Merrill-Palmer Quarterly, 55*(4), 488–515.

Cabanes, J. V. A., & Acedera, K. A. F. (2012). Of mobile phones and mother-fathers: Calls, text messages, and conjugal power relations in mother-away Filipino families. *New Media & Society, 14*(6), 916–930.

Cheong, K., & Mitchell, A. (2015). Kwento: Using a participatory approach to design a family storytelling application for domestic helpers. In J. Abascal, S. Barbosa, M. Fetter, T. Gross, P. Palanque, M. Winckler (Eds.), *Human-computer interaction – INTERACT 2015* (vol. 9298, pp. 493–500). Seattle: Springer International Publishing, Technology & Social Change Group, University of Washington Information School.

Chib, A., Wilkin, H. A., & Hua, S. R. M. (2013). International migrant workers' use of mobile phones to seek social support in Singapore. *Information Technologies & International Development, 9*(4), 19–33.

Cooley, C. H. (1902). The looking-glass self. *O'Brien*, 126–128.

Crabtree, A., Hemmings, T., Rodden, T., Cheverst, K., Clarke, K., Dewsbury, G., ... Rouncefield, M. (2003). *Designing with care: Adapting cultural probes to inform design in sensitive settings.* Paper presented at the Proceedings of the 2004 Australasian Conference on Computer-Human Interaction (OZCHI2004). Brisbane: Ergonomics Society of Australia.

Dalsgaard, T., Skov, M. B., Stougaard, & M., Thomassen, B. (2006). Mediated intimacy in families: Understanding the relation between children and parents. In *Proceedings of interaction design and children 2006* (pp. 145–152). Tampere: ACM Press.

Fivush, R. (2007). Maternal reminiscing style and children's developing understanding of self and emotion. *Clinical Social Work Journal, 35*(1), 37–46.

Fivush, R. (2008). Remembering and reminiscing: How individual lives are constructed in family narratives. *Memory Studies, 1*(1), 49–58.

Fivush, R., Bohanek, J. G., & Duke, M. (2008). The intergenerational self: Subjective perspective and family history. In *Self continuity: Individual and collective perspectives* (pp. 131–143). New York: Psychology Press.

Fivush, R., Haden, C. A., & Reese, E. (2006). Elaborating on elaborations: Role of maternal reminiscing style in cognitive and socioemotional development. *Child Development, 77*(6), 1568–1588.

Fivush, R., Bohanek, J. G., & Marin, K. (2010). Patterns of family narrative co-construction in relation to adolescent identity and well-being. In *Narrative development in adolescence* (pp. 45–63). Boston: Springer.

Forghani, A., & Neustaedter, C. (2014). *The routines and needs of grandparents and parents for grandparent-grandchild conversations over distance.* Paper presented at the Proceedings of the 32nd Annual ACM Conference on Human factors in Computing Systems. Toronto.

Frensch, K. M., Pratt, M. W., & Norris, J. E. (2007). Foundations of generativity: Personal and family correlates of emerging adults' generative life-story themes. *Journal of Research in Personality, 41*(1), 45–62.

Gaver, B., Dunne, T., & Pacenti, E. (1999). Design: Cultural probes. *Interactions, 6*(1), 21–29.

Gaver, W. W., Boucher, A., Pennington, S., & Walker, B. (2004). Cultural probes and the value of uncertainty. *Interactions, 11*(5), 53–56.

Graham, C., & Rouncefield, M. (2008). *Probes and participation.* Paper presented at the Proceedings of the Tenth Anniversary Conference on Participatory Design, Bloomington.

Horst, W., Bunt, T., Wensveen, S., & Cherian, L. (2004). *Designing probes for empathy with families.* Paper presented at the Proceedings of the Conference on Dutch directions in HCI, New York.

Hutchinson, H., Mackay, W., Westerlund, B., Bederson, B. B., Druin, A., Plaisant, C., ... Hansen, H. (2003). *Technology probes: inspiring design for and with families.* Paper presented at the Proceedings of the SIGCHI Conference on Human factors in Computing Systems, Boston.

Kellas, J. K. (2010). Narrating family: Introduction to the special issue on narratives and storytelling in the family. *Journal of Family Communication, 10*(1), 1–6.

Kiser, L. J., Baumgardner, B., & Dorado, J. (2010). Who are we, but for the stories we tell: Family stories and healing. *Psychological Trauma: Theory, Research, Practice, and Policy, 2*(3), 243.

Koenig Kellas, J., & Trees, A. R. (2006). Finding meaning in difficult family experiences: Sensemaking and interaction processes during joint family storytelling. *The Journal of Family Communication, 6*(1), 49–76.

Lim, S. S., & Soon, C. (2010). The influence of social and cultural factors on mothers' domestication of household ICTs–Experiences of Chinese and Korean women. *Telematics and Informatics, 27*(3), 205–216.

Luusua, A., Ylipulli, J., Jurmu, M., Pihlajaniemi, H., Markkanen, P., & Ojala, T. (2015). *Evaluation probes.* Paper presented at the Proceedings of the 33rd Annual ACM Conference on Human Factors in Computing Systems. Seoul.

Madianou, M. (2012). Migration and the accentuated ambivalence of motherhood: The role of ICTs in Filipino transnational families. *Global Networks, 12*(3), 277–295. doi: 10.1111/j.1471-0374.2012.00352.x.

Madianou, M., & Miller, D. (2011). Mobile phone parenting: Reconfiguring relationships between Filipina migrant mothers and their left-behind children. *New Media & Society, 13*(3), 457–470.

McAdams, D. P. (2004). *Generativity and the narrative ecology of family life*. Mahwah: Lawrence Erlbaum Associates Publishers.

McCarthy, J. R. (2012). The powerful relational language of 'family': Togetherness, belonging and personhood. *The Sociological Review, 60*(1), 68–90.

McDougall, Z., & Fels, S. (2010). *Cultural probes in the design of communication*. Proceedings of the 28th ACM International Conference on Design of Communication, ACM, New York, pp. 57–64.

MOM. (2014). Singapore workforce. http://stats.mom.gov.sg/Pages/Singapore-Workforce-2014.aspx. Accessed 1 July 2015.

MOM. (2015). Foreign workforce number. http://www.mom.gov.sg/documents-and-publications/foreign-workforce-numbers. Accessed 1 July, 2015.

Pennebaker, J. W., Kiecolt-Glaser, J. K., & Glaser, R. (1988). Disclosure of traumas and immune function: Health implications for psychotherapy. *Journal of Consulting and Clinical Psychology, 56*(2), 239.

Peterson, B. E., & Klohnen, E. C. (1995). Realization of generativity in two samples of women at midlife. *Psychology and Aging, 10*(1), 20.

Pratt, M. W., & Fiese, B. H. (2004). *Family stories and the life course: Across time and generations*. London: Routledge.

Quek, K. M.-T. (2014). The Evolving challenges of modern-day parenthood in Singapore. In *Parenting across cultures* (pp. 145–161). Berlin: Springer.

Rahman, N. A., Yeoh, B. S., Huang, S., & Yeoh, B. (2005). Dignity overdue: Transnational domestic workers in Singapore. In: *Asian women as transnational domestic workers* (pp. 233–261). Singapore: Marshall Cavendish Academic.

Roberts, J. (1994). *Tales and transformations: Stories in families and family therapy*. New York: Norton.

Seidman, I. (2013). *Interviewing as qualitative research: A guide for researchers in education and the social sciences*. New York: Teachers College Press.

Stone, E. (2004). *Black sheep and kissing cousins: How our family stories shape us*. New Brunswick: Transaction Publishers

Taylor, A. C., Fisackerly, B. L., Mauren, E. R., & Taylor, K. D. (2013). "Grandma, tell me another story": Family narratives and their impact on young adult development. *Marriage & Family Review, 49*(5), 367–390.

Thomas, M., & Lim, S. S. (2011). On maids and mobile phones: ICT use by female migrant workers in Singapore and its policy implications. In J. Katz (Ed.), *Mobile communication: Dimensions of social policy* (pp. 175–190). New Brunswick: Transaction Publishers.

Thompson, E. C. (2009). Mobile phones, communities and social networks among foreign workers in Singapore. *Global Networks, 9*(3), 359–380.

Trees, A. R., & Kellas, J. K. (2009). Telling tales: Enacting family relationships in joint storytelling about difficult family experiences. *Western Journal of Communication, 73*(1), 91–111.

Vutborg, R., Kjeldskov, J., Pedell, S., & Vetere, F. (2010). *Family storytelling for grandparents and grandchildren living apart*. Paper presented at the Proceedings of the 6th Nordic Conference on Human-Computer Interaction: Extending Boundaries, New York.

Wong-Villacres, M., & Bardzell, S. (2011). *Technology-mediated parent–child intimacy: Designing for Ecuadorian families separated by migration*. Paper presented at the CHI '11 Extended Abstracts on Human Factors in Computing Systems, Vancouver.

Wyche, S. P., & Grinter, R. E. (2012). *"This is how we do it in my country": A study of computer-mediated family communication among Kenyan migrants in the United States*. Paper presented at the Proceedings of the ACM 2012 Conference on Computer Supported Cooperative Work, Seattle.

Yeoh, B. S., & Huang, S. (1998). Negotiating public space: Strategies and styles of migrant female domestic workers in Singapore. *Urban Studies, 35*(3), 583–602.

Part II
Intimacies

Chapter 5
Mobile Technology and "Doing Family" in a Global World: Indian Migrants in Cambodia

Ravinder Kaur and Ishita Shruti

Abstract This chapter compares and contrasts the use of mobile and internet technologies among two sets of Indian migrants in Cambodia. One set consists of rural and less educated single male migrants from eastern India, while the other comprises highly educated professionals generally migrating with family from across the country. Education, income levels and the cost of technologies at the destination country shape migrants' access to technologies, with the professionals using more sophisticated technologies and the rural migrants depending more on simpler and commercially available public facilities. We use the trope of "doing family" to explore the transformations in the nature of communication between migrants and various left-behind family members. More frequent and timely communication allows migrants to produce intense affective bonds that regenerate the "family feeling" required to reproduce the family as a transnational corporation of kin. Especially for the rural migrants, ICTs enable faster and more frequent financial remittances, underlining their character as a "currency of care"; additionally, they help strengthen homeland culture and occasionally subvert gender and age hierarchies. Among the professionals, globalised, multilocal families are able to keep in constant touch, mitigating in part the pain of separation.

Keywords International migration • Mobile technologies • Doing family • Intimacy • Remittances

---

R. Kaur (✉) • I. Shruti
Department of Humanities and Social Sciences, Indian Institute of Technology Delhi, Hauz Khas, New Delhi, India
e-mail: ravinder.iitd@gmail.com

Globalisation, Migration and New Communication Technologies

As noted by many scholars, migration has grown immensely over the last several decades (Castles and Miller 2009; Cohen 2008; Faist 2000; Kivisto and Faist 2010). More people are able to migrate to new destinations to seek different kinds of work and lead lives far away from home. This has led scholars to remark that

> The twin processes of globalisation and migration are fundamentally changing the nature of our everyday experiences…forcing a redefinition of intimate and personal aspects of our lives, such as the family, gender roles, sexuality, personal identity. (Giddens 2001, p. 61 in Ziehl 2003 p. 324)

Key to the transformations in this phase of globalisation is the role of technology, especially information and communication technology (ICT). Highlighting its importance, Appadurai (1996) describes what he calls the "post-globalisation world order" as one in which "technology, both high and low, both mechanical and informational, now moves at high speeds across various kinds of previously impervious boundaries" (p. 34). Pointing to its social consequences, Giddens (1990) notes that the revolution in ICTs has facilitated "time–space compression" and that "social life is now ordered across time–space" (p. 64). However, in keeping with the contemporary understanding that technology and society mutually shape each other, Parrenas (2005) points out that "…the compression of time and space in transnational communication is not a uniform condition, but a varied social process shaped by class and gender" (p. 318).

The Transnational Perspective

The nature of international migration has been continuously evolving in recent decades. Migrants who do not become permanently resettled abroad but who spend considerable lengths of time in foreign locations now constitute a considerable proportion of the migration stream. Such migration might also involve being in multiple locations over the life course. As Faist (2000) mentions, in the past, migration meant a radical break with one's place of origin, disruption of social ties and a loss of one's culture. Due to the lack of rapid or affordable transportation, return visits and continuous contact with family back home were difficult, thereby adversely affecting the quality of relationships that could be maintained. Over time, advancements in transportation, the proliferation of communication technologies and growing prosperity have led to the emergence of robust transnational communities that are constantly in touch with home. These changes have led to the emergence of the "transnational perspective" in migration theory that captures the processes and outcomes of interactions between migrants and their homeland. Faist (2010) defines the "transnational social field" as "…combinations of social and symbolic ties and their contents, positions in networks and organisations, and networks of organisations that cut across the borders of at least two national states" (p. 1673).

The transnational perspective in migration studies has the advantage of taking into account both sides of connections and flows (migrants and those left behind), by mapping the networks and channels through which people and resources move (Upadhyay and Rutten 2012, p. 58). These flows produce and shape multistranded social relationships (Burrel and Anderson 2008).

Thus, both migration and new ICTs are reconfiguring people's lives. On the positive side, migration provides fresh economic and social opportunities to voluntary migrants, while ICTs provide easy and affordable ways for migrants to keep in touch with families they have left behind. On the negative side, the social costs of migration cannot be understated, especially its effects on fractured families. One debate in current migration and ICT literature is whether these new technologies are able to alleviate some of the social and human costs of migration and to what extent (Huang et al. 2008; Madianou and Miller 2011; Parrenas 2001, 2005). More broadly, research on the role of ICTs in the lives of families split up by migration is growing steadily with diverse findings on how these new ICTs are shaping or rewriting relationships, challenging or reiterating extant structures and hierarchies. Huang et al. (2008) pose the question of the manner in which the liminality of migrants – "neither here nor there" – might be transformed by ICTs into the simultaneity of "both here and there". More importantly, they point to the need to study the dynamics of this process and its outcomes in diverse locations and under diverse circumstances.

Family, Remittances and ICTs

This paper looks at the role of ICTs, especially mobile phones, in the South–South migration of rural and urban Indians to Cambodia. While many recent studies on mobile telephony and migration have concentrated on female migrants from East Asia, our study focuses on single male rural migrants and migrant families with urban, professional backgrounds. Adopting the framework of "the possibilities of simultaneity" (Huang et al. 2008, p. 7) provided by new ICTs such as mobile phones and computer-mediated communication, we explore two main questions: (1) How do ICTs enable migrants to "do family" across international borders? (2) How does the availability of cheaper and faster means of communication influence and reshape migrants' remittance behaviour? We take the concept of "doing family" from West and Zimmerman's (1987) idea of "doing gender", a performative approach, and argue that migrants and their families employ these technologies to enact gendered familial roles and obligations that achieve a "reinstitution" of the family across borders (see Bourdieu 1998). The continuous acts of doing family facilitated by the new ICTs allow the migrants to produce the intense affective bonds that regenerate the "family feeling" required for the reproduction of the family as a "transnational corporation of kin" while giving meaning to and justifying the separation caused by migration.

We argue that in the case of the Indian migrants in Cambodia who are the subjects of our study, there is a close relationship between "doing family" and remittances. Zelizer (2006) in her work on money and intimacy points out that intimate social transactions coexist with monetary transactions and that such transactions might even have large macroeconomic consequences as in the case of remittances by migrants. In several developing countries such as the Philippines, Sri Lanka, Thailand and India, it is the "family feeling" embodied in monetary remittances that generates large flows of cash which are invaluable in sustaining households and economies. Similarly, McKay notes that economic provisioning is an integral part of emotional nurturing (2007, in Madianou and Miller 2011) and kin and money intertwine in various ways in migrants' relationships. Further, money is not the only form that remittances take: gifts of various sorts also help nurture meaningful social relationships from a distance. In fact, as Bray (2007, p. 40) points out "consumption has become the principal site for the production of meaning and the reproduction of power relations in modern societies" and consumer goods brought or sent by migrants perform multiple functions of sustaining relationships through gifting, display of social status and as signs of successful migration.

Mobile technologies and communications generate new and faster ways of sending remittances, enabling migrants to respond to diverse family needs. In the past, money could not be transmitted as rapidly, or a migrant could not make immediate plans to visit a family member in distress. As our ethnography will later show, responding to emergencies and the speed of such response allows migrants to be more meaningfully and effectively involved in the day-to-day affairs of the left-behind family. Yet, as Tenhunen (2008) remarks, "the new mobile technologies draw from local social cultural and political processes" and cannot act by themselves (p. 517). Different possibilities are afforded by infrastructural, class and regional constraints within which subjects manoeuvre to adapt and shape technologies via networks of kinship, neighbourhood and friendship.

Background: Indian Migrants in Cambodia

The focus of our paper is the technology-based communication practices of two sets of Indian migrants in Cambodia. We refer to one set of migrants as "Mosquito Net Sellers" (MNS): rural migrants who originally came to Cambodia to sell primarily mosquito nets but are now itinerant sellers of a variety of goods in the Cambodian countryside and downtown areas and markets in urban areas. They are natives of eastern India, originating mostly in the district of Gorakhpur in the state of Uttar Pradesh. Theirs can be characterised as chain migration as historically new migrants have followed older ones from the same region. International migration has entered their "calculus of choice" (Hugo 2005, p. 95 in Huang et al. 2008, p. 3) establishing migration as a livelihood and mobility strategy. Kinship and village ties constitute the social capital that enables the movement of males to the capital of Cambodia, Phnom Penh. We call the second set of migrants "Professionals" as they are highly educated Indians who see their migration to Cambodia as a stepping stone on the path of further career mobility and subsequent migration to Western countries. They hold well-paying jobs in various sectors like pharmaceuticals or in international NGOs. In comparison to the MNS, the Professionals originate from diverse parts of India and are more often than not accompanied by their families. They thus form part of the new transnational middle class (Biao 2002; Upadhya 2004).

Methodology

The second author collected ethnographic data on the two groups of migrants in Cambodia from 2008 to 2009. Data was collected through (a) a socio-demographic survey of selected Indian migrants, (b) in-depth interviews with a subset of the first group and (c) participant observation among both groups of migrants. As the second author was living in Cambodia as part of family migration, she occupied the position of an insider with the group of Professionals while she was both an insider and an outsider with the second group, the MNS, by virtue of being from the same native region. Although her education and class position set her above them, she managed to establish a high level of rapport in both cases, and was able to gather detailed ethnographic data over the fieldwork period.

Survey

A respondent survey was conducted with a total of 188 Indian migrants (151 MNS and 37 Professionals, including women). The goal of the survey was to create a database of the socio-economic characteristics of Indian migrants to Cambodia and to enable rapport building with the two migrant groups in order to study their experiences and strategies in South–South migration. English was used to communicate with the Professionals and Hindi with the MNS. The data was collected through personal visits with all respondents, especially the MNS, and also through email communication with some of the Professionals.

Interviews

A smaller group of migrants from both groups was interviewed intensively through open-ended interviews. The sample of MNS varied by duration of stay, age, caste and marital status and the Professionals varied by gender, age, income, locality of residence, occupation, linguistic and regional background, marital status and type of migration (i.e. family or single). In all, 26 MNS (all men) and 25 Professionals (13 women and 12 men) were interviewed. One interview was conducted with the wife of an MNS in Delhi. Most of the interviews were conducted in the respondents' own settings, usually at their domiciles. Some interviews were conducted at workplaces and one was conducted in a restaurant. MNS were also interviewed in groups in their "rooms" or residential accommodations. Throughout the chapter, respondents are referred to by initials such as "PV" or "RV" to protect their identities.

Socio-economic Characteristics of the Migrants

MNS represent a homogeneous group in terms of their occupation in Cambodia, though a few of them have diversified their businesses. In terms of religion, they are mostly Hindu (around 92.7 %) and dominated by castes designated as "backward" by the Indian Constitution (around 66 %). Approximately 64 % fall into the 25–40 age group. Their average monthly income is approximately 100 USD (around 61 % earning between $75 and $100). Among MNS, approximately 48 % had high-school qualifications, 22 % attained less than high school qualifications, and 23 % exceeded high school qualification but fell short of a university degree. Migrants with graduate degrees are a small minority at only 7 %. Although approximately 85 % of the MNS are married, all have migrated to Cambodia without their families.

As previously mentioned, the Professionals form part of the new transnational middle class and their profile is strikingly different from that of the MNS. Though the Professional group is dominated by people aged 25–40 years, around 37 % are above 40 years of age. Around 60 % of the Professional migrants are Hindus, followed by Christians (22 %). In contrast to the MNS, around 94 % of the married Professionals (84 % were married) had migrated along with their families to Cambodia.[1] Unlike most MNS who experienced a sudden move from village to a foreign land, most of the Professional migrants had experienced internal migration before attempting international migration.

Mobile Phone Penetration and Ownership

According to a news report by the Cambodian Information Center (2007), in 2007, the Cambodian mobile phone market had 1.5 million subscribers compared to 4200 fixed-line subscribers with an annual growth rate of about 35 %. This figure rose to 4.3 million in 2009, representing 29 % penetration with a growth rate of 50 %, with nine operators competing with one another (Sharma 2010). As a result, Cambodia

---

[1] Representation of family migration may be high as respondents were mostly approached through female members of the group. However, observation in an Indian restaurants frequented by this groups revealed a considerable number of "involuntary bachelors" in Cambodia, mostly working in the pharmaceutical industry.

became heavily dependent on mobile phones, with landlines becoming a rarity (Sharma 2010). However, international outgoing phone calls from mobile phones were very expensive in Cambodia. Mobitel, one of the most preferred service providers, charged almost one USD per minute for international calls to India. Between late 2008 and early 2009, it introduced a different system, popularly known as "177", in which prefixing 177 with the country code reduced the cost of international calls to only 20 cents per minute. The other option was internet-based phone calls, which were the cheapest option for communication available in Cambodia. Internet cafés provided Yahoo messenger and Skype for international calls. A few internet cafés offered these services for about five cents per minute. Thus, internet-based phone calls became the most preferred mode of communication for the MNS.

India has also witnessed a huge technological advance in telecommunication. According to the Telecom Regulatory Authority of India (TRAI), the total number of telephone subscribers in India was almost 900 million with a total teledensity of around 72 % (2011). This is a big leap considering that in 2006 the teledensity was a meagre 12.8 % and the total number of subscribers was just 130 million (Malik n.d.; Tenhunen 2008). However, the rural–urban divide still persists in India. According to TRAI (2013), out of approximately 900 million subscribers in March 2013, only 38.88 % were rural subscribers. In recent times, rural India has witnessed better growth in both penetration and teledensity from 2010 to 2011 compared to urban India (TRAI 2011).

The use of mobile phones was high among the Indians in Cambodia but with a huge variation between the two groups: among the Professionals, almost every migrant had a handset (which is how mobile phones are referred to in Cambodia), but among the MNS the availability of handsets was restricted to a few powerful and successful migrants referred to as "room leaders".[2] The two groups also varied in terms of their use of communication technology. Though the internet is one of the main mediums of communication for both sets of migrants, modes of use differ. The Professionals have a range of choices – from mobile phone calls to internet-based communication practices such as chatting, emailing and social networking on sites such as Orkut and Facebook. The communication of the MNS, on the other hand, was primarily through telephone calls from internet cafés which offer Skype and Yahoo messenger services. The MNS and their families back home thus fell more into the category of "have-nots" or "information have-less" in a digitally divided world (Cartier et al. 2005; Mannur 2003).

The ownership of mobile phones by MNS depended on many factors such as the success of their business in Cambodia, the number of dependents they had, the amount of savings and their family background. For example, many MNS, although earning a decent wage, did not possess a mobile phone because a large proportion of it was remitted for family expenditure back home. Yet in contrast, some MNS

---

[2] The MNS resided in various one-bedroom apartments in downtown areas of Phnom Penh called "room" by them. Each room had a "room leader" who would be like a "patriarch" of a family. The "room leaders" usually belonged to the dominant caste group of the room, who was also a successful migrant in Cambodia.

might not have been earning very much but owned a handset. Since most of the phones were bought in Cambodia, they did not have Hindi keypads. Consequently, only a few MNS used texting/SMSs as most were not well versed in English. Even among the migrants with high school qualifications, many did not know enough English to text.

Most MNS used mobile phones only for receiving incoming calls. The main reason behind such usage was the high cost of international calls in Cambodia and India. They would simply receive the call and then go to the "booth" (internet café) to make a long phone call. The "booth" operator would dial the number through Skype or Yahoo Messenger and the migrants would talk to their family members for several hours. Most of the migrants had at least one mobile in their family back home, which had been bought with remittance money. Before internet-based calls were introduced, virtual connectivity between migrants and "home" was highly limited for the MNS. Previously, when mobile phone calls were less affordable, they would make calls once a month or during special occasions such as festivals. The calls were of short duration as the respondent quoted below reveals. In comparison with the past, both the length and quality of communication have altered.

> Earlier, when we used to call, it was for a maximum of one or two minutes with the conversation going thus: "Ok. How are you, everything alright?" That's it. Now it is different, we speak for as long as we wish to. (RY)

The important goal was to maintain the link even though not much meaningful conversation could take place. The continuous communication now ensures that home and homeland is no longer just a memory, sustained by occasional contact, but an integral part of the migrants' daily lives (Hiller and Franz 2004).

Back in India, the left-behind families did not experience a gradual process of greater connectivity, that is, from landline to mobile phone, but immediately leap-frogged to mobile telephony. The success of communication via phones and internet, however, remains dependent on the availability of networks and bandwidth wherever the migrants and their families are located. Besides affordability, skills and competencies at both ends were important for the success of communication. The usage of more sophisticated communication technologies reflected differential educational levels, class and status among users. Sometimes, however, the pattern of usage could cut across the class divide. For example, Professional migrants who did not have internet access at home in Cambodia or whose family members in India were not comfortable with the new technologies would also go to the "booth" to make internet-enabled phone calls. These visits were usually for making multiple calls during Indian festivals or if the call was going to be a long one.

Asian Migration and the Family

A major area of investigation regarding international migration centres around the question of how migrants relate to their homeland, focusing mainly on how they maintain family ties and how they create and maintain social capital (Burrel and Anderson 2008). Theorists like Huang et al (2008), Yeoh et al (2005), Osella and Osella (2008) and Gardner (2010) note that in the Asian context, migration does not result in permanent rupture, but the migrating individuals and families stay connected through ties that remain alive within a system of mutual obligations and responsibilities. Basch, Glick-Schiller and Blanc (1994, p. 261) point out that irrespective of the "cultural histories" of the particular group of migrants, in each case (e.g. their Filipino and Caribbean subjects), "kinship has been stretched and reconfigured as families have been extended transnationally".

Lack of permanent rupture from families is also an outcome of the fact that the bulk of Asian migration in contemporary times consists of labour migration with migrants having no intention of settling at their destination, although their migration trajectories may be long and complex (Kesavapany et al. 2006). Among the MNS, only males migrated, leaving behind their wives and children with resultant "transnational families". The conditions for single male migration emerged due to restrictions on women's migration and the cost of relocating with the entire family. In the case of the Professionals, however, single male or female migration was motivated by individual goals and not due to the presence of gender bias or the cost of migration.

"Doing Family" Among MNS

Migration of an individual family member, as argued by Huang et al. (2008), is best captured in the notion of the "transnational corporation of kin". Family ties remain highly valued and the cultural emphasis on the family as a source of support and of social and economic capital remains resilient. The decision to "do family" across border(s) is reflected in what Bourdieu (1998, p. 68) calls "the practical and symbolic work" that is needed to generate "family feeling". He talks of the exchange of gifts, service, assistance, visits, attention and kindnesses that do the work of integration. We examine some of these exchanges, focusing on remittances as a major type of exchange for migrants and other more subtle aspects of doing family across borders via mobile technologies that involve care, emotion and affection which "perpetuate the structures of kinship and family as bodies" (Bourdieu 1998, p. 68).

As noted earlier, new ICTs perform the function of bridging and effectively shrinking geographical distances. Increased frequency of contact and long conversations help in transcending the boundary between "absent" and "present" family members (Giddens 1990; Hiller and Franz 2004). Information exchange has not only become speedier, its content has also grown steadily richer and more time-bound

(Ballard 2003). More recent literature discusses how mobile phones and the internet have changed the dynamic of keeping in touch and have introduced the possibility of "virtual intimacies" (Wilding 2006, in Huang et al 2008) between migrants and left-behind members, whether they are parents, children or spouses (Parrenas 2005). Intimacy emphasises socio-emotional aspects of "doing family" over transnational spaces (Landolt and Wei 2005). The migrants try to make up for their absence through regular communication by phone.

ICTs enable migrants to respond more quickly to emergent or expressed needs of family back home. As revealed in the narrative below, events that earlier evoked a sense of helplessness on the part of the migrant could now be attended to, further strengthening emotional ties with the family.

> My son was running a high temperature for the past few days. My wife started crying over the phone. Then I called up my younger brother and told him to admit my son to a good hospital in Gorakhpur. (PV)

The ease and frequency of phone communication thus achieved two things in this case: it gave an opportunity to ANI (PV's wife) to bargain with her husband for better healthcare for her son and it also gave PV the ability to play the role of the caring and providing father by seeking better treatment for his son. While the gendered appropriation of technology might reify existing gender regimes (as men continue to have greater access), subtle differences get introduced. The mobile affords the wife direct access to her husband, thereby enhancing her power within the joint family. At the same time the husband's role as a provider gets reiterated and his importance in the family is further underlined due to his superior earnings from migration.

Conjugal intimacy, especially between younger couples, has always been very constrained within the Hindu joint family. Mobile communication alters this by allowing couples to have direct and unmediated contact with each other. A respondent, JV, had migrated soon after marriage and his wife was living with his parents. Daily phone communication had helped him maintain emotional intimacy with his wife. As a result, one day, when he received a call from his brother saying that his wife had been hospitalised, he left immediately for India. He was supposed to be helping his boss with a new business but got so distressed at the news that the latter allowed him to go home. The consequences of such actions spurred by instant communications disrupt the social field and create it anew. He was able to sustain intimacy in his long-distance marriage, and at the same time, his travel to take care of her when she was ill allowed his wife to demonstrate to her in-laws the strength of her relationship with her husband, and she gained greater influence in the joint family as a consequence.

In the Indian context, where filial and sibling relationships are often given greater public importance than conjugal ones, telephones were deployed to maintain intimacy between siblings as well (Valentine 2006). Brothers and sisters called back and forth to remain connected with one another – "This was the first time I was away from my sisters on *Rakhi*[3]; we spoke over the phone for 5 hours continuously;

---

[3] Rakhi is an important festival in North India signifying the bond between brothers and sisters.

my youngest sister was also crying and so was I" (JPS). Thus, the expression of emotion which was barely possible in the earlier short, time-bound staccato-paced calls, limited to didactic speech, allows for the retention of the affective richness of relations between family members.

New communication technologies also helped reproduce the native culture among migrants through the correct observance of ritual practices of the household. All major Hindu North Indian festivals like *Navratri*, *Diwali* and *Holi* were collectively celebrated by the MNS. Family members in India would convey many small details of the rituals and festivals, such as their exact date and time according to the Hindu calendar, over the phone. During *Diwali*, they could thus offer *pooja* (prayers) at the ritually determined auspicious time. Forgotten details of various rituals could be conveyed over the phone, thereby ensuring that many more rituals and festivals were observed and binding the migrant closer to both family and his/her native land. The urge for assimilation into the host country's culture lessens because emotional satisfaction can be derived from one's native culture. The back and forth communication over such observances and celebrations thus allowed the migrants to preserve their culture and solidarity at the place of migration.

Mobile phones were also a preferred gift that MNS took home. However, the gift was only given to very close family members or to someone through whom the migrant's status could be enhanced, such as a particular uncle, brother or in-law. As mentioned earlier, even if the gift was for the older parents or uncles, it would be operated mainly by younger people. The ownership of mobile phones also increased the status and power of some wives if they possessed their own handset gifted by the "providing husband". Hence, mobile technology had the potential to chip away at some patriarchal relationships within the joint family.

"Doing Family" Among the Professionals

The context of migration of the Professionals was wholly different from that of the rural MNS and the separation of their urban middle-class families occurred due to very different impulses-the expansion of production sites and movement of capital along with labour that the Professionals were participants in (Sassen 1988). Such migrants are making strategic choices to maximise the capabilities and opportunities of each family member – the husband's, wife's, and even the children's – whether for work or for higher education. Therefore, among middle-class migrants, families are fractured more out of choice than of necessity. Separation from family members is borne as the cost of achieving individual goals. Such families display a pattern in which multiple homes and multiple forms of families are very much a reality (Baviskar and Ray 2011; Beck 1992; Landolt and Wei 2005).

Various forms of transnational families were found among the Professionals in Cambodia due to their multi-migration pattern. We highlight three types of spatially separated families: *first*, those who migrated as a nuclear family and were thus separated upon migration from extended family members such as parents and siblings;

second, families where only one spouse migrated, leaving behind the remaining spouse and the children (bi-local families where the nuclear family is located in two places); and *third*, where a nuclear family was spread across multiple places – multilocal families.

Due to their complex migration trajectories, family members experienced multiple separations and reunifications in their lifetime, and some families remained spatially divided for long durations. For instance, AN's family, comprising himself, his wife and their two sons, moved between Mumbai and Delhi in India, the Maldives, Botswana and Cambodia due to job opportunities and their children's education. Finally all four were located in different countries: the husband in Cambodia, the wife in Botswana, the elder son in India and the younger one in Swaziland. The family was partially reunited when AJ (the wife) moved to Cambodia with her younger son while her elder son moved to Mumbai after completing his studies in Delhi. In another family, the man alone relocated, while his wife and children remained at home in India, which resulted in a bi-local nuclear family. In a third case in which both spouses were doctors (RA and her husband), they moved around between Saudi Arabia, the UK, Cambodia and Tonga, while their children stayed at home in Hyderabad, India. On growing up, the children moved to New Zealand to study and eventually the family became multilocal – a family of five spread across four different countries and three continents – RA in Cambodia (Asia), her husband in Tonga (Asia-Pacific), her older son and daughter-in-law in the USA (North America) and her two younger sons in New Zealand. Yet this spatial separation did not mean that the migrants were disconnected from their families as they adopted different strategies to remain connected. If globalisation has resulted in the spatial rupturing of families, it has also increased the spread of technological advancement which has helped members to remain connected. How the separation is bridged and mediated among the Professionals differs substantially from the MNS who had limited choices. The former were able to exercise a much greater range of choices among communication technologies and practices from mobile phones to chatting, emails and use of social networking sites such as Orkut and Facebook. The technological skills and access of left-behind family members determined the choice of mode of communication. For example, around 40 % (10 out of 25 respondents) had their family members in smaller Indian towns and cities which had limited internet access in 2008. Therefore, migrants with left-behind family members in these places had limited use of internet-based communications such as chatting and communication through video-call platforms such as Skype and Google Talk. Internet-based calls were quite popular in the group until mid-2008, before the major service providers reduced the international phone call rates to India to 20 cents per minute. From mid-2008 onwards, migrants had also started using their mobile phones for making regular calls. However, for special occasions and for calls of longer durations, migrants still went to internet cafés to make calls.

Furthermore, access to the internet at home determined and gendered usage (Mitra 2001). Among the 25 respondents from this group, 50 % either did not have internet access at home or the husband had an office-issued laptop which he would carry to work. Due to the lack of internet or computer access at home, women were dependent on their husbands for communicating with their families back in India. As Skype-based calls were cheaper than telephone calls, women had to wait for their husbands to return home with their laptops in order to communicate with their families via Skype. In families with computers and internet connectivity at home, migrant women dominated the use of the internet in Cambodia. In such families, it was interesting to see how these women negotiated their time and space to chat with their natal family members (*maike wale*) back in India and with friends outside Cambodia. Access to technology allowed them to embrace a more meaningful modernity even if within established gendered hierarchies:

> I generally Skype with my parents during the morning hours, when my husband and kids are not around. Then again in the afternoons when my husband goes back to work after lunch, my son is sleeping and my daughter is still in school. These are the times for networking; I am very frequently on Facebook. I love it. (BH, female)

Communication and the Quality of Life

The most common strategy among Professional migrants to make family separation bearable was to communicate regularly. In some cases, they spoke to their family members almost every day. Regular phone calls or chatting with parents and siblings were also evident among those who had migrated with family. Mediated face-to-face communication platforms such as Skype and Google Talk have transformed the nature and frequency of communication among these educated migrants, reducing the isolation effects of being far away. Skype calls and chatting would determine the daily routine of some of the migrants. For example, RA did not go anywhere in the evenings, as she reserved that time to communicate with her husband or son over Skype. She said, "Every day I repent that we are separated. Only thing is this Skype and these things keep us going, three times we are in touch every day; he calls me". In multilocal nuclear families, communication technology became a primary expenditure which was specifically budgeted for. For example, AN was spending almost 800 USD on various modes of communication while his family was spread across four countries. Those who had internet access at home could in fact reduce their expenditure on mobile calls by talking on "face-to-face" video conferencing platforms.

Marriage remains one of the most significant rites of passage in India and arranged marriage involves much negotiation. The possibility of influencing significant marriage decisions of family members back home is enhanced by the possibility of Skype and Yahoo Messenger communication which make a qualitative difference in how communication happens. Thus, BH's husband was able to help his younger brother with negotiating his choice of spouse with their parents.

> My brother-in-law is planning to get married. Proposals are pouring in. He sends us the photographs over email. He wanted to meet one girl on his own. He told my husband to talk to their father about it. My in-laws are a bit conservative, so they may not allow him to meet the girl. But, my husband can convince them. We are planning to have a conference call with all of them. (BH, female)

Yet such communication could only be effective because of BH's husband's position as an important member of the family, despite his physical absence. His international job and his position as the elder son and primary earner allowed him to negotiate more space in family decision-making rather than being constrained by the availability of technology.

Remitting Money as "Doing Family"

Bringing together the complex threads of globalisation, migration and new communication technologies, we now address the ways in which mobile and other communication technologies facilitate the dispersal of transnational capital and allow individuals to nurture family ties as well as achieve mobility-related goals of migration. Remittances sent by migrants are one of the most important transnational connections between migrants and their left-behind family members, as well as significant symbols of successful migration (Cohen 2011). However, the thematic discussion on remittances has, until recently, been overly economic (R. H. Cohen 2011; Singh 2006; Upadhya and Rutten 2012). Shifting the discourse and pointing to the practical and symbolic work that remittances perform among Asians, Singh et al. (2010) call monetary remittances the "currency of care" (p. 246), locating their significance in relationships of family care, responsibility and security. She also calls it "transnational family money" (p. 250) implying that although the single migrant might be the earner, the capital thus generated is shared by all family members and is considered the outcome of the efforts of collective family strategies and sacrifices in sending a member abroad. Successful migration allows migrants to fulfil many family obligations and exhibit their improved status in local society (Cohen 2011; Ganguly and Negi 2010). Remittances also have the potential of changing intra-household dynamics and altering power equations, including gendered ones, in the receiving household (Cohen 2011; Ganguly and Negi 2010). That people can now make instant monetary remittances is highlighted by Singh (2006, p. 387):

> New technologies, particularly Automated Teller Machines (ATMs), provide the possibility of instant remittances. The use of the internet has also made it easier to send remittances. In many cases the post office has given way to banks, and now to online transfers, for sending money home. The use of a phone-based remittance system for remittances to the Philippines has reduced costs and increased convenience.

Remittances by the MNS and the Professionals are contrasted in many ways. Among the MNS, they formed an important part of the household budget among the left-behind families. In some cases, they were their only source of income. Apart from meeting daily family expenses, remittances from MNS were used for various purposes such as building houses, buying agricultural and nonagricultural property, education of children and younger siblings, financing family rituals and festivals and parents' pilgrimages, repayment of debts and the marriage of siblings and children, especially daughters.

These migrants did not follow any set pattern of sending remittances. The frequency of remittances depended on the needs of the family back home. For example, if there were no alternative sources of income back home, they would send remittances on a monthly basis. Otherwise, they would send money as and when required. Prior to the emergence of new ICTs, the frequency of sending remittances by MNS was lower and short-term, need-based remittances were a rare phenomenon. The migrants used to send money periodically with fellow migrants travelling back to their villages. However, with the spread of mobile telephony in India, the latter has become the preferred route. It ensures that migrants could be approached quickly in times of urgent need and immediate response received. As one of the respondents said, "Whenever there is a need for money at home, I tell VY (MNS respondent who arranges transfer of funds in the village), and he goes to the "booth" and calls up his brother in the village to deliver money to my home".

Among the MNS respondents, their remittance process was dependent on three factors: the social capital base at both ends, the ownership of phones and access to phones. Among the MNS, a few "agents"[4] facilitated the remittances at both ends. Family members in India would call up the migrants to express specific monetary needs. Then the migrant would go to his preferred "agent" in Phnom Penh and ask for a particular amount of money to be delivered to his home. The "agent" would go to a booth and call up his family member, usually a man, on his mobile phone and ask him to deliver the amount to the particular house, and the money would reach the migrant's family within hours. Thus, money could now be delivered more frequently and more rapidly. Before the advent of new communication technologies, such quick delivery of monetary remittances was simply not possible.

When migrant PV's newly bought vehicle was stolen in the village in India, communication between him and his brother was key to ensuring the follow-up with police and the insurance company to retrieve the vehicle. His brother would call PV daily to inform him of the progress of the case and would ask for the money needed to follow up with different agencies. His brother did not have to wait for returning migrants to carry the money and he did not have to borrow money from the money lenders in the village.

Tenhunen (2008, p. 515) argues that technologies are "appropriated" rather than simply "domesticated" through people's practices – daily and institutional – within their contexts. The control of the mobile, between 2008 and 2009, was related to the status of the family members. Therefore, if the family had one mobile phone, the authority to use the phone rested with the person managing the remittances. If remittance money was used for business activities, then financing a phone was very common. Even if the migrant did not own a mobile phone in Cambodia, he would purchase them and gift them to family members back home. In the absence of remittance-related business, the phone was mostly kept with the wives or, in the case of unmarried migrants, by a sibling. Mobile ownership did not follow the patri-

---

[4] Agents were generally those people who had better access to capital (economic, social and cultural) than their fellow migrants. They facilitated migrants' arrival in Cambodia as most of the migrants lacked English language skills required for international travel.

archal hierarchy as it was difficult for the older generation to learn how to operate the phones.

The remittance pattern observed among the Professional Indians was very different from that of the MNS even though there was diversity within this group as well. Single migrants, male or female, sent remittances quite regularly. But those who had migrated as a family did not follow any regular pattern. Adept at using technology, the Professionals transmitted money into their own "Non-resident Indian" bank accounts via online transactions. But sometimes they also took cash home with them. Even the purpose of monetary remittances was quite different for different migrants. For example, very few professional migrants were sending money for monthly household expenditure. Most of their remittances were used for different purposes such as real estate investment, sponsoring education for their children or younger siblings, supporting their parents, paying off debts, sponsoring migration of nuclear family members or saving up for their own marriages, as in the case of single female migrants.

The online transfer of funds/remittances came as a big boon to the Professionals, as they did not have the time to make bank drafts and send them to India. Yet, even these migrants hardly used instant money transfer facilities like Western Union, believing that the transaction charges were very high. Some of them also requested their employers to remit part of their salary to their Indian bank accounts in order to save more. This way they were free from the remittance processes. In the case of those who did not send money regularly, the role of phone calls or chatting was much more important. For example, MO, a respondent, did not send money to his parents on a regular basis, as his father was quite self-reliant. But when his parents needed some extra money, they would request it over the phone, and he would transfer the required amount to his father's account.

Conclusion

Technologies of communication have made the "doing" of intimacy and family life across transnational spaces a reality. Our discussion of mobile and internet technology use among Indian migrants in Cambodia and their left-behind families reinforces the sociological truism that society and technology are mutually shaped. This comparative study of rural and urban migrants shows that while there is clear evidence that communication technologies bridge physical, social and emotional distances, the differences in types of technologies accessed, the purposes for which they are deployed and the extent of usage and success of communication are shaped by a host of diverse factors specific to the stage of development of technologies both at source and at destination, as well as circumstances of individual families and the larger context of community. Actors engage actively with communication technologies in their physical and symbolic dimensions to renew, strengthen and reshape family ties and homeland culture. As in many other studies (see Christensen 2009; Pertierra 2005; Valentine 2006; Wei and Lo 2005), we found that "doing family" was made possible by the new mobile technologies and it generally led to strengthening of affective ties. Affective ties and intimacy were enabled and enhanced between migrant men and their left-behind wives, siblings and parents. Among Professionals, who often had multilocal families, ICTs allowed a family life otherwise denied by location in multiple places and time zones (Christensen 2009). Among the rural migrants, family and homeland culture were reproduced through the use of mobile technologies. A significant difference we found between the two groups was that while the professional urban migrants were able to access technology in the private space of their homes, the rural, poorer migrants accessed it mostly in publicly available facilities which resonates with the popularly held view that publicly available technologies are for "have-nots" (Lee 1999, p. 334). Our findings did not reveal significant negative effects of mobile and internet technologies such as Parrenas' (2005) study of long-distance mothering in which grown up children saw frequent calls by mothers as surveillance. Notably too, our findings on how ICT access might change traditional age and gender equations among families of rural Indians and allow urban globalised families to stick together by "doing family" – materially and emotionally – despite being separated by vast geographical distances are significant. Another contribution of the study is to demonstrate the role of mobile technologies in enabling enhanced use of remittances both as "currencies of care" and as means of upward social mobility.

References

Appadurai A. (1996). *Modernity at large: Cultural dimensions of globalisation.* Minneapolis: University of Minnesota.
Ballard R. (2003). A case of capital-rich under-development: The paradoxical consequences of successful transnational entrepreneurship from Mirpur. *Contribution to Indian Sociology, 37*(1&2), 25–57.
Basch, L., Glick Schiller, N., & Blanc C. S. (1994). *Nations unbound: Transnational projects, postcolonial predicaments and deterritorialized nation-state.* London: Routledge.
Baviskar, A., & Ray R. (2011). *Elite and the everyman: The cultural politics of Indian middle classes.* New Delhi: Routledge.
Beck, U. (1992). *Risk society: Towards a new modernity.* London: Sage.
Biao, X. (2002). *Ethnic transnational middle class information: A case study of Indian information technology professionals.* Paper presented at 52nd annual conference of political studies association (UK) making politics count, University of Aberdeen, 5–7 Apr 2002. http://www.psa.ac.uk/cps/2002/xiang.pdf. Accessed 20 July 2011.
Bourdieu, P. (1998). *Practical reason: On the theory of action.* Stanford: Stanford University Press.
Bray F. (2007). Gender and technology. *Annual Review of Anthropology, 36,* 37–53.
Burrel, J., & Anderson, K. (2008). "I have a great desire to look beyond my world": Trajectories of information and communication technology use among Ghanaians living abroad. *New Media & Society, 10,* 203–224.
Cambodian Information Centre. (2007). Cambodian mobile market is growing at an annual rate of around 35%. http://editorials.cambodia.org/2007/05/cambodias-mobile-market-is-growing-at.html. Accessed 6 Aug 2009.

Cartier, C., Castells, M., & Qiu, J. L. (2005). The Information Have-Less: Inequality, mobility, and translocal networks in Chinese cities. *Studies in Comparative International Development*, Summer, *40*(2), 9–34.

Castles, S., & Miller, M. J. (2009). *The age of migration*. New York: Guilford Press.

Christensen T. H. (2009). 'Connected presence' in distributed family life. *New Media & Society*, *11*(3), 433–451.

Cohen, R. (2008). *Global diasporas: An introduction*. London: Routledge.

Cohen, J. H. (2011). Migration, remittances and household strategies. *Annual Review of Anthropology*, *40*, 103–114.

Faist, T. (2000). *The volume and dynamics of international migration and transnational social spaces*. New York: Oxford University Press.

Faist, T. (2010). Towards transnational studies: World theories, transnationalisation and changing institutions. *Journal of Ethnic and Migration Studies*, *36*(10), 1665–1687.

Ganguly, S. & Negi, N. S. (2010). The extent of Association between husband's out migration and decision making power among left behind wives' in rural India. *ARI working paper series*. www.nus.ari.edu.sg/pub/wps.htm. Accessed 8 Mar 2011.

Giddens, A. (1990). *The consequences of modernity*. Cambridge: Polity.

Giddens, A. (2001). *Sociology* (fourth edition). Oxford: Polity Press.

Gardner A. (2010). *City of strangers: Gulf migration and the Indian community in Bahrain*. Ithaca: Cornell University Press.

Hiller, H. H., & Franz, T. M. (2004). New ties, old ties and lost ties: The use of internet in Diaspora. *New Media & Society*, *6*(6), 731–752.

Huang, S., Yeoh, B. S. A., Lam, T. (2008). Asian transnational families in transition: The liminality of simultaneity. *International Migration*, *46*(4), 3–13.

Hugo, G. (2005). The new international migration in Asia: Challenges for population research. *Asian Population Studies*, 1(1) 93–120.

Kesavapany, K., Mani, A., & Ramasamy, P. (Eds.). (2006). *Rising India and Indians in East Asia*. Singapore: ISEAS.

Kivisto, P., & Faist, T. (2010). *Beyond a border: Causes and consequences of contemporary immigration*. Newbury Park: Pine Forge Press.

Landolt, P., & Wei, W. D. (2005). The spatially ruptured practices of migrant families: A comparison of immigrants from El Salvador and the people's republic of China. *Current Sociology*, *53*(4), 625–653.

Lee, S. (1999) Private uses in public spaces: A study of an Internet Café. *New Media & Society*, *1*(3), 331–350.

Madianou, M., & Miller, D. (2011). Mobile phone parenting: Reconfiguring relationships between Filipina migrant mothers and their left-behind children. *New Media & Society*, *13*(3), 457–470.

Malik P. (n.d.). Policy implications of the digital opportunity index (DOI) analysis for India: Capabilities of measurement and importance of extending DOI to a regional level. University of Delhi and LIRNEasia. http://www.itu.int/osg/spu/digitalbridges/materials/malik-paper.pdf. Accessed 28 Feb 2015.

Mannur, A. (2003). Postscript: Cyberscapes and the interfacing of Diaspora. In E. B. Jana & A. Mannur (Eds.), *Theorizing Diaspora* (pp. 281–290). Oxford: Blackwell.

Mitra, A. (2001). Marginal voices in cyberspace. *New Media & Society*, *3*(1), 29–38.

Osella, C. & Osella, F. (2008). Nuancing the 'migrant experience: Perspectives from Kerala, South India, pp. 146–178. http://eprints.soas.ac.uk/5175/1/koshych_5_osellas.pdf. Accessed 22 Sep 2012.

Parreñas, R. S. (2001). *Servants of globalization: Women, migration and domestic work*. Stanford: Stanford University Press.

Parrenas, R. (2005). Long distance intimacy: Class, gender and intergenerational relations between mothers and children in Filipina transnational families. *Global Networks*, *5*(4), 317–336.

Pertierra R. (2005). Mobile phones, identity and discursive intimacy. *Human Technology, 1*(1), 23–44.
Sassen, S. (1988). *The mobility of labour and capital: A study in international investment and labour flow*. Cambridge, MA: Cambridge University Press.
Sharma, A. (2010). *Cambodia's mobile market growing by over 50%*. TMCnet.com viewed on July 2014 http://www.tmcnet.com/channels/telecom-cost-management/articles/79257-cambodias-mobile-market-growingover-50-percent.htm
Singh, S. (2006). Towards a sociology of money and family in the Indian diaspora. *Contribution to Indian Sociology, 40*(3), 375–399.
Singh, S., Cabraal, A., & Robertson, S. (2010). Remittances as a currency of care: A focus on 'twice migrants' among the Indian Diaspora in Australia. *Journal of Comparative Family Studies, 41*, 245–263.
Tenhunen, S. (2008). Mobile technology in the village: ICTs, culture, and social logistics in India. *Journal of the Royal Anthropological Institute* (N.S.), *14*, 515–534.
Telecom Regulatory Authority of India (TRAI). (2011). Annual report of Department of Telecommunication, Ministry of Communications & IT, Government of India, New Delhi. http://www.dot.gov.in/annualreport/2011/English%20AR%202010-11.pdf. Accessed 20 Sept 2014.
TRAI. (2013). The Indian telecom services performance indicators. http://www.trai.gov.in/WriteReadData/WhatsNew/Documents/Indicator%20Reports%20-01082013.pdf. Accessed 20 Sept 2014.
Upadhya C. (2004). A new transnational capitalist class?: Capital flows, business networks and entrepreneurs in the Indian software industry. *Economic and Political Weekly, 39*(48), 5141–5143.
Upadhya, C., & Rutten, M. (2012). Migration, transnational flows, and development in India a regional perspective. *Economic and Political Weekly, 57*(19), 54–62.
Valentine, G. (2006). Globalizing intimacy: The role of information and communication technologies in maintaining and creating relationships. *Women's Studies Quarterly, 34*(1/2), 365–393.
Wei, R., & Lo, V. (2005). Staying connected while on the move: Cell phone use and social connectedness. *New Media & Society, 8*(1), 53–72.
West, C., & Zimmerman D. H. (1987). Doing gender. *Gender and Society, 1*(2), 125–151.
Wilding, R. (2006), 'Virtual' intimacies? Families communicating across transnational contexts. *Global Networks, 6*(2) 125–142.
Yeoh, B. S. A., Hsiu-Hua, S., Piper, N., Lorente, B. P., et al. (2005). Introduction. In B. P. Lorente, N. Piper, S. Hsiu-Hua, & B. S. A. Yeoh (Eds.), *Asian migrations: Sojourning, displacement, homecoming and other travels*. Singapore: Asia Research Institute/National University of Singapore.
Zelizer, V. A. (2006) *Money, power and sex*. Working paper series 06–009, Princeton Law and Public Affairs.
Ziehl S. C. (2003). Forging the links: Globalisation and family pattern. *Society in Transition, 34*(2), 320–336.

Chapter 6
The Cultural Appropriation of Smartphones in Korean Transnational Families

Kyong Yoon

Abstract Drawing on in-depth interviews with the young-adult children of South Korean transnational families in Canada, this chapter explores how the family is reimagined in the mediated, mobile, transnational communication between family members. In the chapter, the smartphone is examined as an assemblage involving earlier media forms and experiences and is thus contextualised in relation to other information communication technologies (ICTs). In addition, the present study addresses the popular use of the Korean-developed communication app, KakaoTalk, among the transnational family members. Furthermore, it explores how the smartphone engages with the preexisting norms of family communication. The research offers insight into how family interaction is technologically mediated across transnational contexts while questioning the technologically deterministic perspective that overestimates the role of mobile technologies in transnational virtual families.

Keywords Smartphone • Korean transnational family • KakaoTalk • Connected presence • Mobile parenting

As mobile information and communication technologies (ICTs) enhance the connectivity of the family across transnational contexts, forms of family interaction, which were conventionally based upon geographic proximity, seem to be increasingly diversified. In particular, transnational mobility via ICTs enables the "virtual togetherness" of the family (Bakardjieva 2003; Wilding 2006). Transnational communication via mobile technologies has been reported as an essential mode of family communication among various transnational families. Given that the family and household have been considered a foundational unit of the appropriation of new technologies (Silverstone and Hirsch 1992), the transnational reformation of family interaction requires media researchers to rethink the process of technology appropriation. ICTs may no longer be simply domesticated in the family as a locality-based unit, but rather integrated into the process in which the family is reorganised beyond locality.

K. Yoon (✉)
University of British Columbia Okanagan, Kelowna, BC, Canada
e-mail: kyong.yoon@ubc.ca

© Springer Science+Business Media Dordrecht 2016
S.S. Lim (ed.), *Mobile Communication and the Family*, Mobile Communication in Asia: Local Insights, Global Implications,
DOI 10.1007/978-94-017-7441-3_6

The transnational family may not be a novel phenomenon. However, the accelerated process of pursuing overseas education has recently led to a recognisable increase in the transnational migration of members of Asian middle-class families (Abelmann et al. 2014; Finch and Kim 2012). In particular, overseas precollege education of children has emerged as a significant driving force of recent transnational migration in middle-class families in Asia. South Korea (hereafter Korea) was one of the Asian countries in which the precollege study-abroad phenomenon grew quickly throughout the 2000s. The annual number of precollege Korean students attending school overseas – mostly in English-speaking countries, such as the United States (US), Canada, and New Zealand – increased nearly fourfold between 2001 (7,944) and 2006 (29,511) (Korean Educational Development Institute 2013). What may be even more significant than the actual figure is the fact that an increasing number of middle-class Korean families are considering their children's precollege study abroad as a probable option (Finch and Kim 2012). The Korean phenomenon of education-driven transnational families can be explained by a combination of two kinds of "social fever": the traditional "education fever," which defines education as the central duty of the family and educational credentials as a crucial component of the family's social status (Seth 2002), and the recent "globalisation fever," evident since the mid-1990s, which leads Koreans to reap the benefits of acquiring English skills and an overseas education (Park 2011). In this respect, the emergence of these overseas-education-driven transnational families implies the reworking of traditional family values in the transnational context. Sending their children to the West for precollege study is thus seen as one of the emerging "family-based strategies responding to globalisation and educational ambition" (Finch and Kim 2012, p. 489).

The phenomenon of transnational families involves not only the flow of education-seeking children and their parents but also the transnational mobility of the ICTs that families use when on the move. The need for constant, mobile, and mediated communication between transnational family members may facilitate the extensive appropriation of emerging forms of ICTs, such as the smartphone and mobile phone applications (hereafter, apps). Like many other Asian countries, Korea has witnessed the rapid diffusion of mobile ICTs over the past two decades. In particular, the smartphone as one of the most recent forms of personal mobile ICT has been so popular among Koreans that, in the 2010s, the country's smartphone penetration rate has been constantly ranked within the top five in the world (Yonhap News 2013). The extensive use of the smartphone, which is not only a form of mobile telephony but also a platform for various internet-based communication and computing tools (Madianou 2014), may reconfigure the ways in which the family is connected, organised, and imagined. Moreover, this reconfiguration may be even further enhanced when ICTs are appropriated by transnational families (Madianou and Miller 2012).

Given the context, the present study explores how the smartphone is incorporated into the communication practices of transnational families.[1] Drawing on empirical

---

[1] This research was supported by the Social Sciences and Humanities Research Council of Canada.

data in the form of in-depth interviews with the young-adult children of Korean transnational families in Canada, the study examines how the family is reimagined in the mediated, mobile, transnational communication between family members. While the study primarily addresses transnational families' use of smartphones, the smartphone here is not simply defined as an isolated and entirely new form of technological object. It is analysed as an assemblage involving earlier media forms and experiences and is thus contextualised in relation to other ICTs. The smartphone, especially through its various apps, enables users to reengage with various media practices (Gardner and Davis 2013). In this regard, the smartphone reifies "remediation" (Bolter and Grusin 1999) processes in which the memories of earlier media are inscribed. The feature of the smartphone as a technology of remediation illustrates how technology use becomes a complicated process involving various places, users, expectations, and practices. Based on the awareness of these features of smartphone technology, the present study examines how the smartphone is adopted by transnational families in relation to other ICTs. In addition, the study addresses the popular use of the Korean-developed communication app, KakaoTalk,[2] among the transnational family members. Furthermore, it explores how the smartphone engages with the preexisting norms of family communication. The research offers insight into how family interaction is technologically mediated across transnational contexts while questioning the technologically deterministic perspective that overestimates the role of mobile technologies in transnational virtual families.

Literature Review

The emergence and popularisation of mobile ICTs has led to attempts to explore the process and meaning of technology consumption in everyday life. Cultural studies-inspired media ethnographies have provided a vivid picture of the cultural appropriation of emerging technologies (e.g., Hjorth 2009; Horst and Miller 2005; Lim 2005; Madianou and Miller 2012; Wallis 2013). In particular, cultural research exploring the "domestication" of technology (Silverstone and Hirsch 1992) has engaged with a contextualised framework in which technology use can be understood as a dynamic and dialectic process between technology, users, and contexts (e.g., Lim 2008). The domestication approach – which often draws on qualitative research methods, such as in-depth interviews or observation – examines technology in relation to the non-technological aspects of users' lives (Haddon 2011) and thus challenges the prevailing technologically deterministic perspective on new technology (Silverstone 2006).

---

[2] KakaoTalk is an interpersonal communication app, developed by a Korean venture company in 2010. Since its introduction, it has been the most popular communication app among Korean smartphone users. While KakaoTalk was initially recognized as an instant messaging app, its other services such as voice calling, group chat, photo sharing, and social media services have also been popular (Jin and Yoon 2014).

Haddon (2011) underscored that, despite the growing number of empirical studies, the domestication studies that have largely been developed in the European contexts have, until recently, rarely addressed non-Western contexts. Thus, Asian-based research on technology domestication is relatively scarce, with the exception of studies that have been conducted in Japan (Ito 2005; Takahashi 2010), Korea (Yoon 2003; Jin and Yoon 2014), China (Lim 2005; Wallis 2013), and throughout Asia (Hjorth 2009; Lim 2008; Lim and Soon 2010). In addition to its Western-oriented empirical focus, the domestication approach has been minimally extended to transnational contexts with only a few exceptions (e.g., Bonini 2011; Madianou 2014; Madianou and Miller 2012). Thus, the understanding of technology domestication appears to still rely, to a great extent, on "methodological nationalism" (Wimmer and Glick Schiller 2002) and fails to capture a vivid picture of the emerging transnational, mobile, ubiquitous media landscape of the family.

The studies of transnational families' ICT use can also be identified in terms of their theoretical focus; that is, it is within a sociocultural or technological context that such studies frame how the family uses emerging technologies. A group of scholars, who are relatively *socioculturally oriented*, has paid more attention to the role of the social and cultural contexts of transnational family life in technology use (e.g., Clark and Sywyj 2012; Elias and Lemish 2008; Hoang and Yeoh 2012; Madianou 2014; Pearce et al. 2013; Parreñas 2005; Wilding 2006). According to these studies, the transnational family's pattern of and ability to engage in transnational communication via ICTs are influenced by factors such as family members' working conditions and available media resources (Hoang and Yeoh 2012), cultural norms (Clark and Sywyj 2012), premigration histories of media use (Wilding 2006), and generational differences (Elias and Lemish 2008).

In comparison, another group of scholars suggested a relatively *technology-oriented* view; they argued that technological features significantly affect how transnational families use ICTs and the types of ICTs they prefer (e.g., Francisco 2013; Vancea and Olivera 2013). The authors claimed that transnational family relationships tend to be renegotiated by new media's technological features that enable or constrain certain aspects of communication. In particular, the technological infrastructure available to the users at the macro level (Vancea and Olivera 2013) or particular technological affordances of new ICTs, such as their visual components (Francisco 2013), can enhance the intensity and frequency of transnational family communication. Furthermore, ICTs' ability for time–space compression empowers migrants or at least enables them to cope with isolation derived from their marginal social position and separation from their left-behind family members (Uy-Tioco 2007).

However, the aforementioned theoretical – sociocultural or technological – foci of the studies of transnational families' use of ICTs are not necessarily mutually exclusive. They have been articulated with each other in a few recent studies that apply the technology domestication approach in a more contextualized way (e.g., Madianou 2014; Madianou and Miller 2012). For instance, Madianou and Miller (2012) addressed the social context of media users and technological affordances in equal measure. While focusing on technological affordances to explore how particular media forms facilitate certain communication patterns, Madianou and Miller (2012) did not ignore the sociocultural context in which technology is adopted, utilised, and negotiated.

In addition to the need to acknowledge both the sociocultural and technological aspects of transnational families' technology use, the expansion of the empirical scope of media research is required. In particular, the literature on the topic has failed to address a wide range of rapidly emerging technologies and various migrant populations. Above all, seemingly due to the temporal gap between academic research and lived media culture, scholarly literature has not included an extensive exploration of the use of smartphones and their apps in the transnational context. Moreover, as the majority of recent studies of transnational families' media use tends to address low-income migrant workers and their families who are left behind (e.g., Francisco 2013; Hoang and Yeoh 2012; Madianou 2014; Madianou and Miller 2012; Parreñas 2005; Uy-Tioco 2007), middle-class families' ICT use in transnational contexts is relatively under-researched, with a few notable exceptions (e.g., Andreotti et al. 2013).

Given the current state of the research on transnational families' use of ICTs, the present study articulates the sociocultural and technological aspects of ICT use while moving beyond a one-dimensional explanation of technology consumption. In addition, this study's focus on young, education-driven migrants from middle-class backgrounds will be a valuable addition that expands the empirical scope of the literature on transnational families' use of mobile technology.

Methodology

The data analysed in the present chapter is derived from qualitative interviews with 38 young Koreans whose families are separated across transnational contexts. The interviews, which constitute a large project on migrants' use of ICTs in Canada, were carried out in three Canadian cities in the province of British Columbia and Ontario – Vancouver, Kelowna, and Toronto – between February and July of 2014. The participants, who are presented under pseudonyms in this chapter, were aged between 19 and 27 at the time of the interviews and had moved to Canada at the average age of 15. About two-thirds of the participants ($n=25$) were separated from both parents, who remained in Korea, while the remainder ($n=13$) were living with their mothers in Canada. The majority of the participants initially entered Canada as international student visa holders, and 14 respondents acquired permanent residency at the time of entry or later.[3]

The interview questions focused on how the young-adult children of Korean transnational families narrated the process of the adoption and appropriation of

---

[3] These young people's acquisition of permanent residency was enabled by their parents being awarded Canadian residency through immigration programs such as the immigrant investor program or skilled worker program.

smartphones, especially in relationships with their family members. Among the data, those particularly focused on smartphone use for family communication were analyzed. To acquire a better understanding of the process of technology appropriation, the respondents were asked to address their present *and* past media practices, especially for family communication, throughout their migrant lives in Canada. Thus, they were given opportunities to narrate and contemplate both their past and current experiences, although it is noted that such a process relies on participants' personal memories and may consequently involve certain bias and selection. Nevertheless, the reconstructed stories themselves seem to meaningfully reveal their transnational media experiences from their current perspective.

Given the aim of the research to explore mobile communication in transnational families, it may have been helpful to conduct interviews with all the family members rather than with the overseas children only. However, due in part to the practical difficulties encountered when attempting to gain access to all family members living across transnational contexts, the research focused on the young-adult children's present and retrospective narratives regarding their communication with their overseas family members. Despite this limitation, the participants' narratives do reveal how their families' media practices are described and reconstructed, although primarily from the perspective of children who use smartphones extensively.

The examination of interviews, which were recorded and transcribed, involved different phases. The initial coding processes identified repetitiously emerging patterns, and this step was followed by focused coding practices that enabled the empirically based generation of a theoretical perspective (Charmaz 2006). Furthermore, through the interpretive and reflexive reading of the transcripts, the implied meanings of what the respondents said were identified and further situated within the sociocultural contexts of the respondents as middle-class transnational youth (Mason 2002).

Connected Presence in Transnational Families

Transnational families, whose members have to maintain long-distance relationships, tend to adopt and test various forms of ICTs and have thus been described as relatively heavy users and early adopters of new technologies (Madianou and Miller 2012; Parreñas 2005). For the younger members of these transnational families, who had to cope with prolonged separation from their parents, always being online seemed to be the default position for family communication (Madianou 2014). For this reason, a few respondents even felt more comfortable with mediated interaction with their parents than they did with face-to-face interaction. Ara, a 19-year-old undergraduate who had been apart from her father in Korea for 5 years, described how she felt about talking to him via telephone versus in person: "When I call, I tend to talk more. It's more comfortable to talk over the phone rather than talking face-to-face. That may be because we [i.e., my dad and I] have been separated for quite some time." Ara lived with her housewife mother in Vancouver while communicating frequently with her father in Seoul via her smartphone. Her face-to-face contact with her father had been limited to once a year or less on average. Ara's lack of face-to-face communication with her father seemed to be supplemented with various forms of ICTs. In particular, her father regularly used programs such as KakaoTalk, Facebook, and Skype via his laptop, smartphone, or office computer, compared to her mother, who did not have her own mobile phone and only used the home telephone.

The significance of mobile technology was evident, especially to a few respondents who had not had their own smartphones until a relatively late phase of their transnational lives. For example, Minju, a 22-year-old female in Toronto who had been living apart from her family in Korea since the age of 17, was one of the few respondents who were relatively ill equipped with personal ICTs compared to the majority of the respondents. She did not have a mobile (2G) phone or personal computer until her final year of high school and thus had to rely on her homestay family's home computer or telephone for transnational communication during this period. Minju was one of a few respondents who did not own their first smartphones until they were in their twenties. In addition to the lack of ICT availability, there was insufficient time to connect with each other because her parents were both employed full time:

> At first, living overseas was tough ... because I didn't have my family here, and I was young. Things [i.e., ICTs] were so inconvenient back then. I called my family using the homestay's house phone. I didn't have a laptop or a mobile phone at that time. In those early days, my mom and dad called me once a month and we talked over the phone for 30 minutes. That was it. I was so lonely.

The families in the present study adapted to the development of ICTs since they had been transnationally separated. The respondents recalled that, especially before adopting smartphones, they had initially used landline telephones along with prepaid international telephone cards and later internet-based voice communications (Voice-over-Internet-Protocol [VoIP], also known as "internet phones" among the respondents) via home computers or internet-customised telephone handsets. Transnational families' use of different ICTs prior to the emergence of the smartphone was well described by older respondents, such as Chan, a 27-year-old Vancouver-based male who recalled the early 2000s when he first came alone to Canada as a precollege study-broad student:

> There was no Skype in those days [laughs]. To contact my family [in Korea], I would buy and use international telephone cards. I would also email. I used Buddy Buddy [an early Korean web-based messenger] with my friends [in Korea], but my parents used email only [among internet-based tools]. Because of the time difference, I couldn't get responses immediately when using email. Regarding international phone cards, they ran out of funds too quickly. Even if I bought a 10-hour card, the 10 hours would go by too fast. As far as I recall now, those things were very, very inconvenient. [...] These days, I use KakaoTalk [for communicating with my parents] because my parents seem to feel comfortable using it.

As evidenced by Chan's recollection, the smartphone seems to have contributed to considerable changes in the ways in which transnational families communicate. The respondents had their own smartphones, which had primarily been purchased when they were in their mid- to late teens in Canada. The smartphone was incorporated into the rhythm of their everyday lives, as Han, a 24-year-old male university student in Toronto, noted: "As soon as I get up, I check messages on my KakaoTalk. Then, I get music playing on my [smart] phone and get ready to go to school while responding to the overnight KakaoTalk messages." Similarly, Suna, a 24-year-old female university student in Vancouver, stated, "I use my iPhone anytime and anywhere [laughs]. Whenever I'm waiting in line or in traffic, or even when I'm eating … it's easy to use and small to carry. I can carry it wherever I go."

The smartphone offered the young people a mediated copresence with the rest of their family as well as friends left behind in Korea. The sense of "connected presence" (Licoppe 2004) was enhanced by various smartphone apps, such as KakaoTalk, Facebook, and Skype. In particular, by exchanging frequent yet brief "link-up" messages or calls (Horst and Miller 2005) on KakaoTalk, the young people tended to maintain their family ties and sense of belonging. Several respondents also shared their everyday stories, often along with their selfies and emoticons indicating their feelings, with their overseas family members and friends, via KakaoStory, the popular add-on for KakaoTalk users. Namjin, a 27-year-old male who had been with his mother in Vancouver since the age of 14, used KakaoStory to keep his father in Seoul updated about his daily life: "KakaoTalk is easy to use. KakaoTalk has KakaoStory, and so people can easily post their selfies, well … with some notes on them. It's like a good combination of texting and Facebook."

In addition to the pervasive use of KakaoTalk, video calls via Skype on smartphones or laptops seemed to enhance the sense of copresence. In particular, smartphones' built-in cameras as well as webcams on laptops were widely used. As observed in recent studies (Francisco 2013; Hoang and Yeoh 2012), visual technologies are increasingly embraced by transnational families who desire to "actually *see* their family when they are away" (Francisco 2013, p. 9). For some respondents, it was evident, at least during the initial period of their overseas family separation, that any single method of mediated communication – voice call, text message, or video message – could not fulfill their desire for copresence: "Although I would call my mom and dad every day, I still felt somewhat limited. So, I tried Skype as well. Then, the internet phone …" noted Somi, a 22-year-old female who relocated to Canada alone at the age of 15. She recalled that she attempted to make as many contacts with her overseas family members as possible by trying different forms of ICTs while coping with separation anxiety during her adolescence alone in Vancouver: "The most difficult thing was … well, I was young and alone. I had been a kind of child who was extremely closely bonded with Mom but was suddenly left alone. It was so … so very challenging."

The popular use of smartphones among the respondents seemed to especially correlate with the ever-increasing availability of, and need for, mobile internet. At the time of the interviews, the respondents, with a few exceptions, were accessing the internet more via smartphone than computer. Yuri, a 19-year-old female student in Vancouver, explained while pointing to her smartphone, "*This* is often more convenient than *that* [pointing to the interviewer's laptop]. With the laptop, I have to use a mouse, but I can touch the whole screen once with this [i.e., her smartphone]."

Of course, the smartphone did not completely replace or displace earlier ICTs but coexisted with them instead (Madianou 2014). At the time of the interviews, some respondents were still using home-based VoIP for family communication – at least at home – because their parents, who either had no smartphones or were not completely comfortable using them, preferred VoIP, the format of which was highly similar to that of traditional landline phones. Various smartphone apps and instant messaging services were often used along with voice calls via smartphones or VoIP services. Overall, the communication practice of instant messaging was deeply incorporated into the respondents' family interaction, in which the importance and necessity of voice was not necessarily replaced with the practice of text messaging (Horst and Miller 2006). Most respondents used voice calling, text messaging, and video calling supplementally rather than relying on a single form of ICT. For instance, text messaging sometimes functioned as a signal to arrange voice or video calls (Bonini 2011). In particular, the smartphone appeared to offer a platform for easily switching between different forms of mediated communication.

According to the respondents, while a few parents were not completely comfortable using smartphones, most were using them or at least adapting to the technology. The parents did not seem to simply resist or reject emerging technologies. For example, Nara, a 23-year-old female who recently began living with her mother in Toronto after several years of living alone, described how her mother was adapting to the smartphone:

> My mom recently switched to a smartphone [from a 2G phone]. These days, I'm teaching her how to use it. My mom is very pleased to have a smartphone because she can now send Dad [in Korea] photos. Although he lives abroad, they [Mom and Dad] can see each other by sharing photos. My mom used to use text messaging frequently in Korea [via a 2G phone]. However, when she came to Canada, she rarely used text messaging. That's probably because text messaging is more expensive here [than in Korea], and she had to type in English [on her 2G phone in Canada]. But, now she can type in Korean with her smartphone, so she began text messaging although she calls more. Thus, I usually use voice call [on my smartphone] when I contact my mom.

As implied in the case of Nara's mother, the smartphone can offer migrants a sense of, and resources for, transnational connection, which enables them to move beyond cultural and linguistic barriers and reestablish a connection with their home countries.

Despite transnational families' enhanced connectivity via mobile ICTs, it is uncertain how effectively mediated interaction compensates for the lack of face-to-face interaction. In the present study, several respondents questioned the sense of virtual togetherness afforded by ICTs. Mediated interaction did not necessarily fulfill the young people's need for proximity-based emotional ties with the family. As some respondents described, mediated family interaction occasionally caused miscommunication and created distance between family members. For example, when asked to compare communication with her parents via smartphone and face-to-face, Yuri, a 19-year-old female in Vancouver, noted, "I prefer to talk face-to-face. It's difficult to fully express what I really want to say via phone calls and texts. However, if I see Mom, I can look her in the face and know how she responds." Moreover, some respondents did not necessarily view mediated interaction as being as meaningful as face-to-face conversation. For example, according to Nuri, a 25-year-old female in Toronto,

> I went back [to Korea] and stayed for about six months last year after graduation. I realised why I had been feeling a little empty. It was the family. It was so good being there [in Korea] with the family. However, I also realised that I had changed since leaving Korea; I thought, I might have a greater sense of belonging to Canada now.

Nuri, a recent graduate who hoped to acquire Canadian permanent residency in the near future, had been communicating frequently with her family members in Korea since her entry into Canada at the age of 14. She had been using various smartphone functions extensively, such as KakaoTalk, iPhone's FaceTime, and Skype, to maintain contact with her family on a daily basis. However, she noted the absence of her physical proximity to her family as a missing part of her adolescence. Nuri's account implies, while being increasingly taken for granted, the virtual togetherness of transnational families maintained by mediated interaction feels incomplete, especially when compared with face-to-face togetherness. This finding echoes the previous observation that mediated communication between transnational families involves certain costs, such as emotional distance (Lan 2003).

Mobile Parenting and Family Norms

The smartphone was a resource not only for young people but also for their parents. The respondents recalled the occasions on which their parents had kept track of the little details of their everyday routines. The mobile internet and various communication apps enabled on smartphones appeared to intensify the micromanagement or even surveillance of the users by others in networked contact (Madianou 2014). In the connected presence allowed by smartphones, it seemed difficult to opt out of being online continually. Such "mobile parenting" or "mediated parenting" has been reported in previous studies (Chib et al. 2014; Lim 2008; Ling and Yittri 2006; Madianou and Miller 2012; Uy-Tioco 2007), although the specifics of parenting may be different, depending on cultural contexts.

Transnational mobile parenting was often the extension of preexisting parental control over ICTs during the respondents' pre-immigration period since they had been allowed, for a restricted time, to use the internet and/or mobile phone. However, since their migration to Canada, the respondents had been released, to some extent, from social and parental pressures due to their physical distance from their parental homes. Even for those who lived with their mothers in Canada, parental control over ICT use tended to be more relaxed than before migration. Of course, this does not mean that parental supervision of children's ICT use disappeared in the transnational context. Rather, it seems that the focus of parental monitoring with regard to children's ICT use was transformed from the direct control of ICT use to indirect yet mobile control through smartphones (Chib et al. 2014). In this process of mobile parenting, preexisting cultural norms seemed to reemerge.

First, the role of preexisting family norms was observed in obligatory family ties between parents and children via mobile communication, which has been addressed in previous media studies of Asian families (Lim 2008; Madianou and Miller 2012; Yoon 2003). In particular, the use of the Korean-developed popular app KakaoTalk between the respondents and their parents appeared to reaffirm the reciprocal yet obligatory process of family interaction. Similar to other communication apps, KakaoTalk notifies message senders as soon as the receiver has seen the message, and thus, children seemed to feel obliged to respond promptly to their parents. In this regard, KakaoTalk might work as a "parent app" (Clark 2012) with which parents can keep track of their children and thus be assured of their safety via mobile communication.[4] Overall, KakaoTalk was extensively used in family contexts, in contrast to other communication apps, such as Facebook, which were widely used with networked contacts. KakaoTalk's circle of "Friends," tended to represent contacts who were highly bound by (physical and emotional) locality. Since KakaoTalk allows only those who share their smartphone numbers to be included in each other's contact list, an individual's KakaoTalk contacts tend to comprise the people whom he or she has met in person and can call via telephone at least occasionally. This system of a phone number-based small circular network seems to distinguish KakaoTalk from some other communication apps that tend to accelerate the economy of size. That is, KakaoTalk contacts are neither exclusively online nor networked to the public. In addition, the young people in the study tended to send their Korean friends and family members KakaoTalk's various cute emoticons and stickers. In response, their parents sometimes, if not often, sent them emoticons as well. For the transnational KakaoTalk users, the KakaoTalk-specific emoticon was an essential communication tool, which was not simply a supplement to texts. The expression of users' emotions via KakaoTalk's humorous and cute emoticons seemed to mediate any tensions that might occur in distant, mediated communication.

In the respondents' accounts, many parents – especially mothers – wanted to frequently confirm their children's daily routines from a distance, as also observed in previous studies (Chib et al. 2014). Jihee, a 19-year-old female who had been living alone in Toronto as an international student for over five years while her parents had remained in Korea, described the way in which the smartphone kept her connected to her mother, which, at times, made her feel obliged to respond. She explained how her mother kept track of her via the smartphone and the popular smartphone app KakaoTalk to ensure that she was all right:

> As usual, one day, my mom sent KaTalk [i.e., KakaoTalk] messages to me and then made KaTalk voice calls, but I didn't answer. When I got back to her two hours later, she was

---

[4] The parents' extensive use of KakaoTalk reflects the fact that it has been the most popular app among Koreans since its launch as a free smartphone app in 2011 in Korea. The number of subscribers (100 million) is already double that of the Korean population in 2013, which signals the app's popularity even outside of Korea. KakaoTalk has been widely used across generations, which distinguishes it from other social network apps, such as Facebook (Kim and Shin 2013). KakaoTalk's particular technological features have been considered an important factor in its popularity (Clayton 2013). In particular, among other merits, the coexistence of older and newer media forms in its simple interface design, which may easily appeal to parents, might be an important factor contributing to the wide use of KakaoTalk among Korean transnational families.

wailing. I felt bad, so I try to reply to her quickly these days. [That time,] my mom [in Korea] contacted me before she went to bed, but I didn't know that I got those messages because it was daytime here [in Canada], and I was in quite a noisy place. My mom said she was worried that I didn't reply quickly.

Second, mobile parenting tended to be gendered in its pattern, as the traditional gender roles of breadwinning fathers and nurturing mothers were by and large maintained. With the exception of a few cases in which both father and mother were employed full time, most respondents relied on the financial remittances of their left-behind fathers during their stay in Canada. The preexisting mode of gendered parenting appeared in the respondents' accounts of the relatively caring, intimate mother compared to those of the strict, distant father. In particular, for the respondents who were separated from their fathers in Korea yet lived with their mothers in Canada, the fathers were described as both physically and emotionally distant figures. For instance, Yuri, a 19-year-old female undergraduate who with her mother had moved to Vancouver 6 years ago, described how she communicated with her parents:

It's not quite necessary to contact Mom on the mobile phone because she is with me [living together in Vancouver]. Well, in regard to Dad [in Korea] ... he has been away for over six years now, so I am no longer likely to talk to him about every single detail of my life, which I still talk to my mom about.

Their emotional distance from their fathers and intimacy with their mothers was especially evident among several female respondents and their mediated communication with their parents. Even for respondents whose parents were both in Korea, their mediated communication with their mothers tended to be more frequent than with their fathers. In addition, some respondents preferred to contact their fathers in Korea via written communication using the KakaoTalk app or emails, whereas they contacted their mothers in Korea via voice calls along with KakaoTalk messaging. Based on a few young people's accounts, mothers, rather than fathers, preferred voice calls via home telephones, smartphones, or internet phones over text messaging. In those cases, the mothers were relatively less comfortable with new technology, while the fathers seemed to have high accessibility to various ICTs at work and home. In this regard, the fathers were described by most respondents as being "busy with work" or relatively "traditional." As Nuri, a 25-year-old female in Toronto, stated:

Dad is really busy all the time [...] My dad is somewhat traditional, so he doesn't do much Skype or KakaoTalk [...] I often talk with my family [i.e., each of my family members via media], but it is rare for all my family members to be together on the phone or Skype. [It happens] just a couple of times per year, I suppose.

Owing to the relative emotional distance between fathers in Korea and children in Canada, mothers, whether in Canada or Korea, played the role of moderators of the communication between overseas children and other family members. This role of mothers as observed in the present study echoes the findings of the previous studies of Korean families' ICT use. For example, Lim and Soon's (2010) ethnographic study found that Korean mothers used ICTs not only for monitoring their children but also for enhancing mother–child bonding, while some mothers appropriated ICTs for improving relatively distant father–child relationship commonly observed in patriarchal family cultures. As shown in the examples of mediated, mobile parenting in the present study, the smartphone, along with other ICTs, served to maintain the bonds between separated family members. However, this does not necessarily mean that smartphone-mediated communication substantially transforms the preexisting cultural norms in which the role of parents remained largely gendered (Madianou 2014).

Conclusion

The present study has explored the role of the smartphone in the Korean transnational family phenomenon driven by the children's precollege study abroad. It has revealed that smartphone-mediated communication is increasingly incorporated into the Korean transnational families' lives, and thus, always being online becomes the ordinary pattern of communication for those families. This chapter's empirical study contributes to the literature on transnational families' use of ICTs in three key ways.

First, given the lack of investigation into smartphones in transnational families, the present study offers valuable empirical data on how the smartphone's technological features, such as its enhanced mobility, connectivity, and storytelling functions, allow transnational family members to negotiate not only their distant relations but also different options of being connected. The smartphone's role as a platform on which numerous communication apps converge seemed to play a significant role in redefining family communication in transnational contexts, as it allows its users to switch easily between different communication media and methods (e.g., visual, iconic, and textual methods). In the present study, among various forms of ICTs and smartphone apps, the Korean-developed communication app KakaoTalk was commonly used by Korean transnational families. Through its internet-mediated voice calling, text messaging, group chat, and journal-keeping services, KakaoTalk appeared to enable the Korean transnational families to be online constantly. The app also contributed to the extensive use of smartphones not only by young people but also by their parents.

Second, this study's focus on middle-class transnational families distinguishes it from previous studies' predominant attention to low-wage migrant workers and their left-behind families. In contrast to "forced" migrant workers, the middle-class Korean families in the study seemed to more willingly engage in family separation in pursuit of the children's "global" cultural capital, which consists of English ability and academic credentials. While the migrant workers' and their families' mediated communication tended to be significantly constrained by relatively poorer material and technological resources (Law and Peng 2008), the transnational children of middle-class background in this study were not similarly encumbered but instead manifested cultural negotiation between the mediated, individualised communication practices and the conventional, face-to-face practices of family communication. In addition, as most respondents – especially those who had been separated from both parents – were able to return to Korea for every school vacation or at least once a year, their virtual family togetherness was regularly supplemented by face-to-face togetherness, unlike low-income migrant families who had to go through prolonged separation.

Third, the present research offers insights into how the existing framework of technology appropriation drawing on domestication theory can be revised. The increasing transnational family phenomenon challenges the significance of the physical boundary of the home as the everyday place of technology appropriation. For most respondents who spent their adolescence at the homestay family's house or a rented or owned condominium with their mothers, who relied on the breadwinning fathers' remittances from Korea, their physical and emotional attachment to the household in Canada seemed tenuous. Partly due to the temporality of the home, the transnational young people in this study – especially those who had been separated from both parents – tended not to own and use many sedentary, household ICTs, such as big-screen, satellite televisions, at their residences in Canada; rather, they heavily utilised personal and portable ICTs, such as the smartphone. The young people's fragile attachment to the overseas household and the extensive use of mobile technologies implies a complex process of technology appropriation in transnational contexts. The phenomenon of transnational families involves the highly individualized management of family time, space, and norms, while the members' desire for physical togetherness and conventional family relations, such as gendered parenting, are not replaced with virtual togetherness. However, with the emergence of the smartphone as a gateway to various modes of communication apps, the individualized mode of overseas living and the nostalgic desire for home seem to coexist.

The transnational families' cultural appropriation of smartphones can be referred to as a "transnational domestication of technology." As domesticity itself may be largely dislocated in the era of mobile technologies (Morley 2003, p. 450), the family is reimagined in the moral economy of the transnationally mobile household, and in this regard, smartphones seem to offer different user strategies. This understanding helps us move beyond the locality-based imagination of the family and its technology appropriation. The transnationalisation of the family itself requires a cross-national understanding of technology and thus "methodological transnationalism." In this regard, the chapter suggests that media studies itself needs to be mobile so that transnational media users can be better traced beyond their sedentary nodes.

References

Abelmann, N., Newendorp, N., & Lee-Chung, S. (2014). East Asia's astronaut and geese families: Hong Kong and South Korean cosmopolitanisms. *Critical Asian Studies, 46*(2), 259–286.

Andreotti, A., Le Gales, P., Fuentes, M., & Javier, F. (2013). Transnational mobility and rootedness: The upper middle classes in European cities. *Global Networks, 13*(1), 41–59.

Bakardjieva, M. (2003). Virtual togetherness: An everyday-life perspective. *Media, Culture & Society, 25*(3), 291–313.

Bolter, J. D., & Grusin, R. (1999). *Remediation: Understanding new media*. Cambridge, MA: MIT Press.

Bonini, T. (2011). The media as 'home-making' tools: Life story of a Filipino migrant in Milan. *Media, Culture & Society, 33*(6), 869–883.

Charmaz, K. (2006). *Constructing grounded theory*. New York: Sage.

Chib, A., Malik, S., Aricat, R. G., & Kadir, S. Z. (2014). Migrant mothering and mobile phones: Negotiations of transnational identity. *Mobile Media & Communication, 2*(1), 73–93.

Clark, L. S. (2012). *The parent app: Understanding families in a digital age*. Oxford: Oxford University Press.

Clark, L. S., & Sywyj, L. (2012). Mobile intimacies in the USA among refugee and recent immigrant teens and their parents. *Feminist Media Studies, 12*(4), 485–495.

Clayton, T. (2013). Why the largest social network in 2015 won't be Facebook, and will be from Asia. http://insights.wired.com/profiles/blogs/why-the-largest-social-network-in-2015-won-t-be-facebook-and-will?xg_source=activity#axzz3CCLYzO8A. Accessed 1 Sept 2014.

Elias, N., & Lemish, D. (2008). Media uses in immigrant families: Torn between "inward" and "outward" paths of integration. *International Communication Gazette, 70*(1), 21–40.

Finch, J., & Kim, S.-K. (2012) Kirŏgi families in the US: Transnational migration and education. *Journal of Ethnic and Migration Studies, 38*(3), 485–506.

Francisco, V. (2013). "The Internet is magic": Technology, intimacy and transnational families. *Critical Sociology, 41*(1), 173–190.

Gardner, H., & Davis, K. (2013). *The app generation: How today's youth navigate identity, intimacy, and imagination in a digital world*. New Haven: The Yale University Press.

Haddon, L. (2011). Domestication analysis, objects of study, and the centrality of technologies in everyday life. *Canadian Journal of Communication, 36*(2), 311–323.

Hjorth, L. (2009). *Mobile media in the Asia-Pacific: Gender and the art of being mobile*. London: Routledge.

Hoang, L. A., & Yeoh, B. S. (2012). Sustaining families across transnational spaces: Vietnamese migrant parents and their left-behind children. *Asian Studies Review, 36*(3), 307–325.

Horst, H., & Miller, D. (2005). From kinship to link-up: The cell phone and social networking in Jamaica. *Current Anthropology, 46*(5), 755–778.

Horst, H., & Miller, D. (2006). *The cell phone: An anthropology of communication*. Oxford: Berg.

Ito, M. (2005). Mobile phones, Japanese youth and the replacement of social contact. In R. Ling & P. E. Pedersen (Eds.), *Mobile communications: Renegotiation of the social sphere* (pp. 131–148). London: Springer.

Jin, D. Y., & Yoon, K. (2014). Reimagining smartphones in a local mediascape: A cultural analysis of young KakaoTalk users in Korea. *Convergence: The International Journal of Research into New Media Technologies*, Online first. 1354856514560316.

Kim, Y. H., & Shin, S. (2013). SNS user demographics. KISDI Report. 26 Dec 2013.

Korean Educational Development Institute. (2013). *Korean educational statistics services*. http://kess.kedi.re.kr/. Accessed 4 July 2014.

Lan, P. C. (2003). Maid or madam? Filipina migrant workers and the continuity of domestic labor. *Gender & Society, 17*(2), 187–208.

Law, P. L., & Peng, Y. (2008). Mobile networks: Migrant workers in southern China. In J. E. Katz (Ed.), *Handbook of mobile communication studies* (pp. 55–64). Cambridge, MA: The MIT Press.

Licoppe, C. (2004). Connected presence: The emergence of a new repertoire for managing social relationships in a changing communication technoscape. *Environment and Planning D, 22*(1), 135–156.

Lim, S. S. (2005). From cultural to information revolution: ICT domestication by middle-class Chinese families. In T. Berker, et al. (Eds.), *Domestication of media and technologies* (pp. 185–204). Maidenhead: Open University Press.

Lim, S. S. (2008). Technology domestication in the Asian homestead: Comparing the experiences of middle class families in China and South Korea. *East Asian Science, Technology and Society: An International Journal, 2*, 189–209.

Lim, S. S., & Soon, C. (2010). The influence of social and cultural factors on mothers' domestication of household ICTs: Experiences of Chinese and Korean women. *Telematics and Informatics, 27*(3), 205–216.

Ling, R., & Yttri, B. (2006). Control, emancipation, and status: The mobile telephone in teens' parental and peer relationship. In R. Kraut, M. Brynin, & S. Kiesler (Eds.), *Computer, phones, and the internet: Domesticating information technology* (pp. 219–234). Oxford: Oxford University Press.

Madianou, M. (2014). Smartphone as polymedia. *Journal of Computer-Mediated Communication, 19*(3), 667–680.

Madianou, M., & Miller, D. (2012). *Migration and new media: Transnational families and polymedia*. London: Routledge.

Mason, J. (2002). *Qualitative researching* (2nd ed.). London: Sage.

Morley, D. (2003). What's 'home' got to do with it? Contradictory dynamics in the domestication of technology and the dislocation of domesticity. *European Journal of Cultural Studies, 6*(4), 435–458.

Park, J. S.-Y. (2011). The promise of English: Linguistic capital and the neoliberal worker in the South Korean job market. *International Journal of Bilingual Education and Bilingualism, 14*(4), 443–455.

Parreñas, R. (2005). Long distance intimacy: Class, gender and intergenerational relations between mothers and children in Filipino transnational families. *Global Networks, 5*(4), 317–336.

Pearce, K. E., Slaker, J. S., & Ahmad, N. (2013). Transnational families in Armenia and information communication technology use. *International Journal of Communication, 7*, 2128–2156.

Seth, M. J. (2002). *Education fever: Society, politics, and the pursuit of schooling in South Korea*. Honolulu: University of Hawaii Press.

Silverstone, R. (2006). Domesticating domestication: Reflections on the life of a concept. In T. Berker, M. Hartmann, Y. Punie, & K. Ward (Eds.), *Domestication of media and technologies* (pp. 229–248). Maidenhead: Open University Press.

Silverstone, R., & Hirsch, E. (Eds.) (1992). *Consuming technologies: Media and information in domestic spaces*. London: Routledge.

Takahashi, T. (2010). Myspace or Mixi?: Japanese young people's engagement with social networking sites in the global age. *New Media & Society, 12*(3), 453–475.

Uy-Tioco, C. (2007). Overseas Filipino workers and text messaging: Reinventing transnational mothering. *Continuum: Journal of Media & Cultural Studies, 21*(2), 253–265.

Vancea, M., & Olivera, N. (2013). E-migrant women in Catalonia: Mobile phone use and maintenance of family relationships. *Gender, Technology and Development, 17*(2), 179–203.

Wallis, C. (2013). *Technomobility in China: Young migrant women and mobile phones*. New York: New York University Press.

Wilding, R. (2006). "Virtual" intimacies? Families communicating across transnational contexts. *Global Networks, 6*(2), 125–142.

Wimmer, A., & Glick Schiller, N. (2002). Methodological nationalism and beyond: Nation–state building, migration and the social sciences. *Global Networks, 2*(4), 301–334.

Yonhap News. (2013). *South Korea tops smartphone penetration rate in 2012*. http://english.yonhapnews.co.kr/news/2013/06/25/90/0200000000AEN20130625003000320F.HTML. Accessed 10 Aug 2014.

Yoon, K. (2003). Retraditionalizing the mobile: Young people's sociality and mobile phone use in Seoul, South Korea. *European Journal of Cultural Studies, 6*(3), 327–343.

Chapter 7
Empowering Interactions, Sustaining Ties: Vietnamese Migrant Students' Communication with Left-Behind Families and Friends

Becky Pham and Sun Sun Lim

Abstract As globalisation continues unabated, migration in general and student migration in particular have intensified worldwide. Mobile communication technologies are important links between migrant students and their left-behind family and friends. This chapter seeks to highlight the complex relationships between the students' migrant status and their technology use, as well as between technology and the family in Vietnamese transnational households. This chapter presents contextualised accounts of three Vietnamese migrant students' media use over a two-week period, drawing data from a one-week media monitoring exercise, a one-week media deprivation exercise, semi-structured interviews and daily media diaries. The study found that the Vietnamese migrant students appropriated a variety of communication technologies to connect with their home country, which helped to energise family interactions, sustain family ties and facilitate parental and sibling mediation, thereby supporting bonding within Vietnamese transnational families. Moreover, the technologies also helped the students to build social capital with their left-behind friends in Vietnam.

Keywords Migrant students • Mobile communication technologies • Left-behind families • Left-behind friends • Media diaries • Media deprivation • Vietnam

---

B. Pham (✉)
National University of Singapore, Singapore
e-mail: beckypham2108@gmail.corm

S.S. Lim
Department of Communications and New Media,
National University of Singapore, Singapore
e-mail: sunlim@nus.edu.sg

© Springer Science+Business Media Dordrecht 2016
S.S. Lim (ed.), *Mobile Communication and the Family*, Mobile Communication in Asia: Local Insights, Global Implications,
DOI 10.1007/978-94-017-7441-3_7

Introduction

Students constitute a growing proportion of the global migrant population. With the intensification of globalisation and the expansion of air travel, more people are crossing borders everyday. As of 2013, more than 230 million people lived outside their home countries, while more than 700 million migrated within their countries (World Bank 2013). Migrating for the purpose of education is rapidly rising. Two million tertiary students studied abroad in 2000, with that figure doubling to four million in 2012 (UNESCO Institute of Statistics 2014). Our study distinguishes between short-term exchange students and long-term foreign students by referring to the latter as migrant students. Exchange students visit host institutions overseas to study for brief periods for cultural exposure and not for academic qualifications. These overseas sojourns are therefore likely to take less planning and preparation and involve minimal academic pressure, with no requirement for long-term cultural integration in the host country. In contrast, migrant students study overseas in search of academic qualifications that they cannot access at home so that they can upgrade themselves and perhaps settle in the host country after graduation to tap more attractive career prospects. Many also strategically choose destinations that offer more opportunities for long-term residency or citizenship after graduation instead of returning to their home countries (Baas 2014; Mazzarol and Soutar 2002). Hence, we feel that the term 'migrant students' is more appropriate for referring to international students of this ilk.

Migrant students contribute significantly to their destination countries, making higher education an increasingly important sector for the economies of those countries. For example, international students contributed $24 billion to the US economy in 2012/2013 (NAFSA 2013), while the Australian economy received just under $14 billion in 2011 (ACPET 2013). Moreover, during their stay in the host country, migrant students may work part-time, participate in social activities or may even become long-term residents after graduation. Thus, they engage in cross-cultural exchange and collaboration while broadening the host country's talent pool. Student migration therefore has considerable social implications and warrants close academic investigation.

Set against this global backdrop, this chapter focuses on Vietnamese migrant students in Singapore. As demand for international higher education increases, Singapore has long exploited its strengths, such as its English-language environment and high standards of education to recruit more students from overseas, thereby establishing itself as a learning hub of Asia and raising the contribution of the education sector to the national gross domestic product (GDP) (Yeoh and Lin 2012). With its proximity to Vietnam and unrivalled reputation for quality education within Southeast Asia, Singapore is one of the top destinations of choice for overseas education for Vietnamese students (Clark 2013). Indeed, Vietnamese students constitute one of the biggest groups of Asian international students in Singapore and numbered an estimated 7000 as of 2011.

According to Wood and King (2002), media and migration are 'two richly interdisciplinary fields of study' (p. 1) that greatly overlap. This chapter aims to offer insight into how Vietnamese migrant students domesticate mobile communication technologies to contact their left-behind families and friend, and what roles such communication plays in maintaining these relationships. As mobile communication technologies act as important links between the students and their family despite the geographical distance, this study seeks to highlight the complex relationships between the students' migrant status and their technology use, as well as between technology and the family in Vietnamese transnational households. It will do so by offering an ethnographic account of their daily lives in Singapore, and how mobile communication is interwoven with their routines, activities and interactions.

Technology Domestication by Families

Technology domestication theory is grounded in the creation of the home (Silverstone et al. 1992, p. 17) sensitising us to how technology is used in the context of everyday life. However, the daily rhythms of the household constitute one's microworld within the larger society, and everyday life encompasses the dialectic between globalising and localising forces (Lie and Sørensen 2002). Given their life situation, migrant students' daily existence inhabits this very nexus. Hence, this chapter explores Vietnamese migrant students' domestication of mobile communication technologies within their everyday life interactions with their host country, as well as with their left-behind families in technology-mediated spaces such as phone calls and virtual environments that are not confined to the physical area of their original households.

Many studies have shown how migrants, especially migrant workers, appropriate communication technologies, most importantly the mobile phone, to build and maintain connections with their left-behind families and friends for the purpose of having a sense of belonging and seeking emotional support as they try to adapt to the new environments of the host countries and the drudgery of their working life (Chib et al. 2013; Lang et al. 2010; Thomas and Lim 2011). With regard to migrant students, they have also been found to utilise communication technologies to keep in touch with their home, especially thanks to the revolutionised and highly reliable mobile phone- and internet-based platforms such as mobile phone calls (Cemalcilar et al. 2005; Constantine et al. 2005; Kline and Liu 2005), instant messages (Kline and Liu 2005; Lim and Meier 2012), emails (Kline and Liu 2005) and social network sites (Hjorth 2007; Lee et al. 2012; Lim and Meier 2012).

A subset of this growing body of literature specifically deals with how migrants appropriate communication technologies to fulfil their familial duties, creating the phenomenon of *transnational mothering* in transnational families. Filipina domestic workers and nurses in the United Kingdom (UK) used video calls, text messages and social media sites such as Facebook to perform their traditional duty as a caregiving parent despite geographical distance and different time zones. They checked their children's daily activities, helped the children with homework and reminded the children of medication to monitor their upbringing just as they could have done if they had been physically at home (Madianou 2012; Madianou and Miller 2011). The fulfilment of a transnational mother's role with the help of communication technologies also holds true for Filipina workers in the United States (US) (Uy-Tioco 2007), Latina workers in the United States (Hondagneu-Sotelo and Avila 1997) and Filipina and Indonesian workers in Singapore (Chib et al. 2014), although mobile phone call bills did put a strain on these domestic workers' financial situation (Madianou 2012; Thomas and Lim 2011). Madianou (2012) also found that Filipino migrants in the United Kingdom monitored their children by signing in to their children's Facebook and email accounts to check their activities, while Chib et al. (2014) discovered that Filipino and Indonesian migrants in Singapore added their children as friends on Facebook and then monitored the children's status and photos.

The technology domestication framework by Silverstone et al. (1992) posits that the household adopts information and communication technologies (ICTs) from the larger formal economy and attaches private meanings to them, thereby transforming them into symbolic values of the household. Such technology domestication processes connect the personal/household economy to the public/formal economy or, in other words, creates the household's 'moral economy' in relation to the public sphere (Silverstone et al. 1992). Hirsch (1992) conducted an ethnographic case study of a British family which revealed how the family's decision to adopt a technology did not depend on the inherent nature of the technology but on the relationships and tensions among family members. Another study by S.S. Lim (2008) showed how communication technologies were an 'indispensable' part of the middle-class Chinese and Korean families' routines and reflect the cultural values of parents–child distance, as well as the important *guanxi* (Mandarin for personal relationships) and *cheong* (Korean for feelings of kinship for family and friends) maintenance. Lemor's study (2006) on communication technology domestication in single parents' households showed that the media was highly relevant to the family and its individuals' practices. As these households changed, their media domestication and especially the monitoring of their children's media consumption also changed. Going through separation and divorce, the single parents experienced financial instability, which limited their choices but increased their control of what forms of media their children could watch. These single parents also had difficulty adjusting to and negotiating with the other parents' media consumption versus their desired ways to monitor the children's media use, which then became tensions that influenced parent–child relationships.

While technology-based familial obligation fulfilment has been well studied among independent, married and adult migrant workers. However, the ways in which younger, single migrant students who are experiencing emerging adulthood act out their roles as a child to their transnational families from afar have not been thoroughly examined. We aim to examine the transnational family phenomenon from the perspectives of migrant children, rather than migrant parents who have been often studied in past literature (see Chib et al. 2014; Hondagneu-Sotelo and Avila 1997; Madianou 2012; Madianou and Miller 2011; Uy-Tioco 2007).

Hence this chapter aims to answer two research questions:

1. How do Vietnamese migrant students appropriate mobile communication technologies into their daily life to communicate with their left-behind families and friends?
2. What roles do mobile communication technologies play in sustaining Vietnamese migrant students' relationships with their left-behind families and friends?

Methodology

We employed three research methods: media diaries, semi-structured interviews and media deprivation to exploit the advantages of all three methods in a complementary fashion. Ethical approval for our research protocol was sought and granted from our institution. Twenty Vietnamese migrant students at a large state university in Singapore were recruited to participate in this study using purposive sampling to capture a range of profile characteristics in terms of age, gender and length of stay in host country Singapore. All of them were studying in Singapore under the local government's scholarship scheme. For each participant, we tracked his/her media ICT use over a two-week period. In the first week, the students' communication activities were monitored with daily media use diaries to understand how they used ICTs for mutual communication with their families and/or friends in Vietnam. The diary took the form of an email questionnaire that was sent to them at the end of each day. The questionnaires comprised both structured and open-ended questions where they were asked to reflect on various aspects of their media use. The students were interviewed face-to-face after the first seven days. In the second week, the students participated in a media deprivation exercise where they were instructed to cease usage of all the ICTs that they typically used to communicate with their families and/or friends in Vietnam and to stop accessing news and information relevant to Vietnam and their hometown, regardless of whether the news source was from Vietnam or not. If the participants accidentally found themselves coming across any piece of news or discussion relating to Vietnam, or to their families and friends back home, they had to immediately stop reading the news and/or refrain from joining in the discussion. No temporary deactivation of social media accounts or phone account was required of them. The purpose of the deprivation exercise was to simulate the condition where migrant students could not access any information about their home country. Apart from this restriction, their ICT use would still proceed as normal. Participants were advised to inform their families and friends in advance of their participation in this exercise. During the second week, the students were again asked to write daily diary entries and reflections on their feelings and experiences of being unable to communicate with their left-behind families and/or friends. At the end of the second week, subjects were interviewed for the second time. Although the interviews were conducted in Vietnamese since it was our participants' first language, they were also free to express their opinions in English if they wished. In light of the relatively prolonged duration of the study and the inconvenience participants had to endure under the deprivation condition, each participant was given an SGD100 book voucher as a token of appreciation.

Findings

To present a more contextualised and in-depth account of the students' technology use, this chapter will present narratives of the lives of three students over the two-week period. These three students' experiences were selected because they represent the broad range of profiles across our sample in terms of the ICTs used to connect with people back home, their communication practices and their family types.

Nhung

A science major, Nhung was 20 years old and had lived in Singapore for one and half years at the time of the research. Originally from Ho Chi Minh City, she came to Singapore to pursue undergraduate studies, following in the footsteps of her elder brother who had also migrated to Singapore for university several years before. Like any migrant student, she had to manage her budget carefully and would tap into her dormitory's Wi-Fi network to access free internet-based services such as Skype and Facebook via her smartphone, laptop and tablet. She would do so even on the go, such as when commuting or attending classes, again accessing free Wi-Fi where available. By assiduously using such free services, she could keep her communication budget low without compromising on the frequency of her communication.

As a consequence, Nhung could communicate with her family (and even extended family) regularly. In the first week, her media diaries showed that she contacted her parents on five different days, her aunt on one day and her cousin on another, mainly to keep all of them informed about her well-being while seeking updates from them as well. She did not speak to her family about anything specific. Conversations were mainly about her studies, daily activities, relationships with friends in Singapore or anything else that could help her feel less homesick. As for her left-behind friends, she had one close friend in Vietnam whom she contacted on two different days to mutually share news on daily occurrences in their lives. Nhung was also very active in using Facebook as a continuous and indirect means to get updates from her left-behind families and friends (Table 7.1).

In communicating with people back home, Nhung selected the appropriate communication channels based on the receivers' technological skills and access. As her parents had basic internet skills but were not avid users, they were not always online. So she would have to call them by mobile phone to ask them to go online to receive her Skype calls:

> Only when I feel the need to talk directly [to my parents], will I use phone calls. Otherwise I will message them on Facebook, or comment [on Facebook]. For Skype, when I need to talk for a long time, I will use video calls to talk for a long time without incurring costs.

Besides the functionality that such technology afforded, they facilitated valuable emotional scaffolding that comforted and nourished Nhung, especially during times of distress. She tended to turn to her parents when she wanted to share stories of how she was coping in Singapore, rather than to her friends in Vietnam or in Singapore, because she believed that her peers would be facing the same issues she was. Her communication with her parents was therefore crucial in helping her to relieve stress:

7 Migrant Students' Communication with Left-Behind Families 115

Table 7.1 Nhung's week 1 media diary

Day	Communication with left-behind family		Communication with left-behind friend(s)	
	Discrete	Continuous	Discrete	Continuous
Thurs	Called her parents on their mobile phone to ask them to go online and then they talked via Skype video calling, discussing her new room on campus	Read Facebook status updates, viewed Facebook photographs on her family members' Facebook profiles	Chatted with her friend about her new room on campus via Facebook messenger	Read Facebook status updates, viewed Facebook photographs and read the news that her friends shared on their Facebook profiles
Fri	Video called her parents via Skype to talk about daily occurrences		None	
Sat	Called her parents to go online and then they talked via Skype video calling about daily occurrences		None	
Sun	Called her parents to go online and then they chatted via Facebook messenger about daily occurrences Chatted with her cousin via Facebook messenger		None	
Mon	Her aunt asked how she was doing via Facebook messenger		None	
Tue	None		None	
Wed	Her parents briefly checked on her via Facebook messenger		Her friend asked how she was doing via Facebook messenger	

Every time I finish talking to my mother [over Skype], I am relieved of my sadness and annoyance because as a student staying away from home, I have just migrated to a new place and most of the friends are international students, so it's hard to integrate well [into the local culture] right after I came here. So when I call her, I feel much better. Having my parents to talk to makes it better.

Indeed, she experienced the full weight of this sentiment during the deprivation condition of the second week. Due to the absence of emotional support from her parents and friends, she found that she could not relieve her stress and, subsequently, became more temperamental:

> I found that there were times [during the second week] that I was more hot-tempered than I normally am. Even my friends here... They asked me 'Why are you so easily irritated these days?' (laughs)

To cope with the situation, she tried interacting more with her friends in Singapore and participating in co-curricular activities. But she felt that those alternatives could only fill the time and help her cope with the media deprivation temporarily and that there was no substitute for communication with her family back in Vietnam:

> When I did not contact my home, I had time to participate in other activities. So I joined a dance group at the place that I'm living at, and I felt very happy. I also signed up to participate in [a] Chingay [class]... [But] often I felt pretty annoyed because there were many times in the day when I had many things that I wanted to share with my mother, to tell my mother so she knows what I have been doing but I could not contact her, so I felt very annoyed.

Besides these discrete communications, Nhung also kept in touch with family and friends via continuous communications such as viewing one another's Facebook updates. She was 'friends' with her family members on Facebook, thus allowing both parties to view one another's social media profile pages for updates at their own convenience. This was a useful supplement to their frequent calls and allowed them to share other aspects using different media such as shared news reports and photographs. However, even as such mutual 'monitoring' had its comforts, it also presented unexpected difficulties. Notably, Nhung recounted how she had once unintentionally given her mother the impression that she did not care about her through her Facebook use:

> One time I called my mother to talk to her on the phone and we argued a little about something. I don't recall what that thing is. But then my mother posted something on her Facebook page. I did not notice that post and I did not 'like' it. One day, I called home. My father picked up the phone and told me that I had made my mother very sad, made her feel like I did not appreciate her anymore because I did not 'like' her post on her Facebook after that argument. My father said that my mother has not been able to sleep because I did not 'like' her Facebook post.

Furthermore, the constant bond forged by mutual monitoring could at times be oppressive when it veered towards surveillance. For example, Nhung felt resentful when her mother intruded too much into her life through their daily communication habits:

> Actually, there were a few times that I went out with my friends and came home late, and called my mother late. So my mother was irritated, like 'Why do you hang out so late?' At that time, I was not very happy either. There was a day when she said, 'when I did not see you do anything on Facebook, I'm afraid you disappear, or go somewhere, or something'.

While she found such experiences irritating, she and her mother never raised it as an issue to be settled and she merely saw them as annoyances she had to live with as part and parcel of the constant connectivity. She did not seek to assert greater independence or to actively remind them that she was an adult in her own right.

Indeed, her parents saw the ICTs as an excellent avenue by which to continue parenting her from a distance. Although Nhung herself seldom brought up any Vietnam-related news she had read during her their Skype sessions, her parents would diligently keep up with news from Singapore and use news reports that they found distressing to caution her against falling prey to online scams. In so doing, her parents were remotely keeping a watchful eye on her, to approximate as far as possible the situation of being there with her physically.

It was also through social media such as Facebook that Nhung got to keep in touch with her friends in Vietnam to share daily experiences or simply to catch up. She valued such online interactions for both emotional and practical reasons:

> I think in the future this [relationship with her left-behind friends in Vietnam] can bring benefits, such as, there are relationships that are always good to keep, the more friends the better, always. But for now, I do not see any benefits but I feel happy when I can help my friends and keep in touch.

The internet was Nhung's only source of Vietnam-related news such as trending news stories in Vietnam, celebrity and entertainment news, and she was not as interested in Singapore-related news. To Nhung, the Vietnam-related news she read served as excellent conversation topics when she interacted with Vietnamese friends both in Vietnam and in Singapore. Her exposure to Singapore-related news was also via the internet, but she admitted that visiting Vietnam-related news websites had already become a habit formed long before she moved to Singapore and that she often found herself unconsciously visiting Vietnam-related news websites much more frequently than those regarding Singapore.

Van

Twenty-three-year-old Van, an engineering major and originally from Ho Chi Minh City, had lived in Singapore for three and a half years for undergraduate studies and was an only child. At the encouragement of her parents, she came to Singapore for a better education and more career opportunities. Her diary reflected that she contacted her parents on five different days and communicated with three friends in Vietnam through short conversations on five different days during the first week of media monitoring, also to update them about her well-being and receive their news just like Nhung. Unlike her friends who were adept at using the internet, her parents were not. Hence, Van had to rely on affordably priced international calling cards to keep in touch with her parents. These cards cost SGD$28 for approximately 5 hours of talk time. Due to her financial difficulty, Van restricted herself to buying only one card to call home per month. If she ran out of calling time towards the end of each month, she would deliberately talk less on the phone with her parents. She was also less active on Facebook compared to Nhung (Table 7.2).

Table 7.2 Van's week 1 media diary

Day	Communication with left-behind family		Communication with left-behind friend(s)	
	Discrete	Continuous	Discrete	Continuous
Thurs	None	None	Friend 1 wished her a happy birthday via Facebook	Read Facebook status updates, viewed Facebook photographs and read the news that her friends shared on their Facebook profiles
Fri	Called her father via mobile phone to receive updates from home		Friend 2 briefly chatted with her via Facebook messenger Friend 3 briefly chatted with her via Facebook messenger	Read Facebook status updates, viewed Facebook photographs and read the news that her friends shared on their Facebook profiles
Sat	Called her parents via mobile phone to talk about family matters		Friend 2 briefly chatted with her via Facebook messenger	Read Facebook status updates, viewed Facebook photographs and read the news that her friends shared on their Facebook profiles
Sun	Called her parents via mobile phone to share with them stories about her internship in Singapore		Friend 2 briefly chatted with her via Facebook messenger Friend 3 briefly chatted with her via Facebook messenger	Read Facebook status updates, viewed Facebook photographs and read the news that her friends shared on their Facebook profiles
Mon	Called her parents via mobile phone to talk about family matters		None	None
Tue	None		None	None
Wed	Called her parents via mobile phone to talk about family matters		None	None

Although Van could not benefit from free, unlimited Skype services the way Nhung did, she made the most of the calling cards and, similarly, received tremendous emotional support from these phone calls:

> Being heard by my parents [over the phone] is being cared for. Well, I don't have the physical care from my parents. Through their listening to me, their sharing with me in times of difficulties or the happiness I experience when I live here [in Singapore], I feel like I still receive their care.

Van said the feelings of concern were mutual. Just as her parents worried about her, she too was concerned about them. So she always felt a sense of duty to remain contactable so as to give her parents peace of mind. Even when they called her when she was at her busiest, she always made it a point to pick up the phone and ask them to call back later, rather than leaving it as a missed call. Indeed, remaining contactable at all times was a key constituent of her overall sense of well-being:

> I will feel more at peace about how my family members are living at home, I can focus more on my studies [if I can contact them when I want to]… I wouldn't have to think, to have to question how my parents are doing, but just focus on my studies.

With the loss of connectivity with her families during the deprivation condition, Van suffered from anxiety and frustration, causing her to lose concentration in studying and working:

> I felt quite worried after…. day 5, day 6 [in the second week of media deprivation]. When I worked, I lost my concentration because… I always felt like calling home to see if there was anything going on at home, I also did not want my parents to worry for me when I am staying here, because I wanted them to know what I was doing, how well I was doing, or what happened to me. I felt that both sides were worried about each other. Asian people like us have something like a premonition when we break something. Before this, if I break something, I will be very worried, I will call my home immediately. Last week [when I was not allowed to contact my parents], I had a cut on my finger, and I could not call my home [so I felt frustrated about it].

Nevertheless, Van did derive some benefits from the deprivation condition. She felt that she learnt to be more emotionally independent and be more active in reaching out to Singaporean friends:

> [The deprivation condition] is one way for me to see if I can survive without calling my parents. I think that [no communication with my parents during the deprivation week] is also a positive thing because we will have to support ourselves and be on our own later on. When our family members are no longer by our side, we will have to be more and more emotionally independent. […] [Hanging out with Singaporean friends during the deprivation week] helps me adapt better to Singapore because I joined many activities that I have never done with Vietnamese friends before.

Like Nhung, Van read online Vietnam-related news more often than Singapore-related news, simply because her friends on Facebook were mostly Vietnamese, and they tended to share such news. She also kept in touch with her friends in Vietnam for future networking opportunities, as she was not entirely confident that she could live in Singapore permanently:

> Because I can never fully be a Singaporean, it is very likely that I will return to Vietnam sooner or later (laugh).

Nam

Having lived in Singapore for more than eight years, Nam's experience differed considerably from those of Nhung and Van. At 24 years old and originally from Hue City in the middle of Vietnam, Nam, a communication major, was also the oldest participant in our study. He had been studying in Singapore since secondary school

Table 7.3 Nam's media diary

Day	Communication with left-behind family		Communication with left-behind friend(s)	
	Discrete	Continuous	Discrete	Continuous
Wed	His younger sister called him via VoIP to talk about her exam grades	Read Facebook status updates, viewed Facebook photographs on his younger sister's Facebook profile	None	Read Facebook status updates, viewed Facebook photographs and read the news that his friends shared on their Facebook profiles
Thurs	None		None	
Fri	Called her younger sister via mobile phone, asking her to go online on Facebook messenger to have a brief chat with him		Friend 1 asked him some information about Singapore's education system	
Sat	None		Friend 2 and Friend 3 wished him a happy birthday via Facebook	
Sun	None		None	
Mon	His younger sister chatted with him via Facebook messenger to ask for a new year gift		Talked about his girlfriend with his two close friends via WhatsApp chat group	
Tue	Called his parents via mobile phone to discuss some issues about his hometown in Vietnam		None	

and stayed on for university education. He was the eldest child, with one younger sister in Vietnam. During the first week, Nam contacted his parents once, his sister four times and five of his friends on three different days. Nam also actively used Facebook to keep updated on happenings in Vietnam (Table 7.3).

While his sister was comfortable with using Skype, voice over internet protocol (VoIP) and social media like Facebook to interact with him, his parents could depend only on mobile phone communication:

> My dad knows how to use the internet but my mom doesn't know. He knows about emails, Facebook, documents, YouTube. But if I tell him to save a page or save an image, as in print the screen, he wouldn't know. He just knows how to browse the internet, but with techniques like opening a new tab, he's a bit slow. My sister is very good at it however. But my mom is totally clueless about it. She just needs a phone.

As the eldest son, Nam felt a strong sense of responsibility towards the family. Unlike Nhung and Van who called home primarily to seek (and offer) emotional support, Nam often used calls with his parents to participate in decision-making processes about the family's finances and relationships with their neighbours. This allowed him to remain deeply involved in family matters and to feel like he had a considerable voice in the household even though he had been away for close to a decade. He made a conscious effort to uphold this independent, adult demeanour so that even when he was stressed and needed a boost in morale from chatting with his family, he would share his personal issues in subtle and understated ways:

> I think my parents could understand what I want to say through the way I talk to them [over the phone]. For example, if I say, 'Today I am very busy', then they would know that I am very stressed. I don't have to say things explicitly like, 'I love you' or 'You love me' or something like that. I call home every time I am stressed, but I will not tell my parents about my stress.

He also extended this sense of duty towards his younger sister – whom he described as a well-behaved, lively but impressionable eight-year-old. He actively played his older brother role, even using Facebook to monitor his sister's online activities from Singapore. When he noticed his sister posting something inappropriate on Facebook, he would speak to her directly and offer advice:

> In real life, my parents can supervise my sister, but they can't do it online. Thus I feel that I have some responsibility in it. I feel that I'm contributing to the development of my family [by monitoring my younger sister from afar]. If my sister develops into a very good person, I would feel proud. [In the second week of media deprivation] I could not see my sister's newsfeed [on Facebook], I didn't know what she was doing, so I felt a bit out of control. [...] Like, if she writes something wrong [on Facebook] but a lot of people 'like' it [and I cannot monitor her], she will think that it is right [and will continue to post inappropriate content].

By casting a brotherly eye over his sister from a distance, Nam could compensate for his parents' limited internet skills and continue to play the roles of supportive brother and involved son, building the family's moral economy in this extension of their domestic space. Furthermore, his sister seemed to take well to his remote supervision as she voluntarily shared with him her daily activities and always accepted his advice for her day-to-day issues.

The import he accorded to this role could be discerned during the second week of the study when the media deprivation condition was in place. Nam realised that he had forgotten that his sister's birthday was during that week and was angry with himself for overlooking that fact when he had agreed to participate in the study. Nevertheless, he voluntarily chose to continue with the research after careful discussion with the researchers. In the interview at the close of that week, he shared that he had felt very guilty and miserable throughout the deprivation period because he believed that sending birthday wishes to one's family members was an important expression of love and care and that, ultimately, his family was his top priority in life.

In addition to connecting with his left-behind family members, Nam had two close friends in Vietnam whom he contacted regularly. As he had been away from Vietnam for such a prolonged period, his networks of left-behind Vietnamese friends were much more limited compared to Nhung's and Van's. Yet Nam said he still saw his friends in Vietnam as 'future investment' and 'potential business partners' if he should return to Vietnam to start a company. While Nhung and Van showed more interest in Vietnam-related news, Nam was equally interested in both countries' news because he felt that while Vietnam-related news gave him information that could influence the well-being of his left-behind family, Singapore-related news would better prepare him for a career in Singapore after he graduated from university.

Discussion

Together, the three vignettes reveal the specific roles that mobile communication technologies play in connecting Vietnamese migrant students to their left-behind families and friends.

Empowering Interactions and Sustaining Ties

Communication technologies clearly provide efficient and convenient continuous connectivity between the students and their left-behind families. Thanks to these technologies, the students are always 'connected', allowing them to easily update themselves on news of their families, inform their families about their lives in Singapore, stay in touch with left-behind friends and also to keep abreast of news about Vietnam. The students could use these technologies to fulfil their roles as children to their families from afar, thereby alleviating the guilt that they could not at home and giving them a sense of belonging since migrant students are often seen as 'strangers' and 'interlopers' rather than as 'future citizens' in the host country (Sidhu 2011).

With the loss of connectivity under the deprivation condition, they suffered anxiety and frustration due to their inability to check on their families' safety and well-being, causing them to lose concentration in studying and working. They came to realise the acute value of connectivity or 'the positive emotional sense that comes from feelings of staying in touch' with important people in their life (Romero et al. 2007, as cited in Wyche and Grinter 2012). The emotional void that they temporarily experienced led them to be stressed or even grumpy towards their friends in Singapore. To cope with the situation, the students tried socialising more with their friends in Singapore and participate in more co-curricular activities. But they felt that these alternatives afforded only fleeting relief and that their communication with their families back home was simply irreplaceable.

However, the strong ties could also be seen as oppressive, especially when remote parental supervision teetered on the edge of surveillance. While the continuous connection and updates enabled by social media offered their parents unobtrusive glimpses into their lives overseas, they also facilitated unwelcome parental interference, consistent with the findings of Madianou (2012) and Chib et al. (2014). Useful as these communication technologies might be in connecting the parents and their children, they were also the only clues for the students' left-behind families to form a superficial and partial picture of their well-being and daily activities in Singapore. Furthermore, with no mutual understanding of how such communications were to be handled, the students found their online actions and omissions misinterpreted, as in the case of Nhung failing to 'like' her mother's Facebook post. In other words, communication technologies were not simply the conduit but also the content of communication between the students and their loved ones, which could lead to magnified expectations of such communication platforms and thus unintentional misunderstandings between communicating parties.

Building Potential Social Capital with Left-Behind Friends

The students were found to mainly use internet-based communication channels to maintain the relationship with their young and tech-savvy friends in Vietnam so that they could offer and receive help when necessary. This connection was a fundamental building block of their social network. The students we studied often received requests from friends in Vietnam to help them buy certain goods in Singapore and bring them back on their trips home. In other cases, friends from back home would also consult them about living and studying in Singapore as some shared similar aspirations. In return, these left-behind friends would reciprocate by delivering things from Vietnam if they happened to visit them in Singapore. This mutual exchange of favours as well as their regular online communication lubricated their long-distance friendships. Over time, they helped the migrant students build an expanded social network back home – one that they planned to tap should they return home eventually (as seen in other studies such as Biswas 2014; Gupta et al. 2014). Although the students only saw the potential of this social network rather than having already experienced benefits, they were fully aware of the mobility and uncertainty in a migrant's life and, hence, attempted to establish and sustain transnational relationships.

Conclusion

The three vignettes above provide contextualised accounts of these Vietnamese migrant students' use of communication technology for communication with left-behind family and friends. Highly mobilised and tech-savvy, they make the most of available communication technologies to expand the domestic space of their individual households. They strategically employ devices such as laptops, mobile phones and calling cards, along with internet-based services such as Skype,

Facebook and WhatsApp, to develop a personalised suite of communication technologies that are best suited to their own and their families' needs, budgets, lifestyles, competencies and constraints. Within this technologically extended domestic space, parental, child, sibling and friendship obligations can be fulfilled, and relationships can grow and not be allowed to atrophy.

The moral economy (Silverstone et al. 1992) of every household can therefore be sustained despite the geographical distance, with parents still actively exercising oversight, children seeking parental affirmation while displaying filial obedience and siblings demonstrating brotherly/sisterly love and support. By appropriating various communication platforms, the students attach symbolic value from their context to these technologies. As they encounter acculturation challenges during their overseas stints, these communication technologies offer a much-needed and greatly treasured connection between themselves and left-behind families and friends. The constant communication and emotional scaffolding help them make sense of their developing identities in the host country, translating into a more tolerable adaptation process. The true value of such familial support was drawn into sharp relief when they underwent the media deprivation condition and experienced distress and sadness at the loss of a source of comfort that they had grown accustomed to and, indeed, reliant upon. The question remains, however, as to whether the students would have developed greater independence and emotional maturity without the constant virtual presence of their parents in their lives overseas. This issue may serve as the springboard for future studies.

Although there is a growing body of research related to migrants and their use of communication technologies, studies on migrant students and specifically those of Vietnamese origin are scant even though they rank ninth worldwide in the number of 'mobile students' (UNESCO Institute of Statistics 2014). This chapter has helped to correct this deficit by studying the communication between Vietnamese migrant students in Singapore and their left-behind families and friends. It has also shed more light on the phenomenon of transnational families by offering the perspectives of migrant children with left-behind families, broadening our understanding beyond the experience of migrant mothers with left-behind children that has dominated previous studies (see Chib et al. 2014; Hondagneu-Sotelo and Avila 1997; Madianou 2012; Madianou and Miller 2011; Thomas and Lim 2011; Uy-Tioco 2007). As well, it has employed a novel media deprivation approach to enable a better grasp of the implications of the presence (and absence) of communication technologies in the lives of migrants.

However, no study is without its limitations. First, the media deprivation exercise took place in the students' natural, uncontrolled setting, making it difficult to enforce the students' strict adherence to the deprivation instructions, although we sought to encourage compliance through the token of appreciation, coupled with regular reminders. Second, to minimise the burden on participants, the media diaries required them to commit only 20 minutes of their time every day, which may have led some subjects to put minimal effort into reflecting on their daily technology use. Future research that adopts the media deprivation approach may wish to take into account these concerns.

References

ACPET. (2013). *Economic contribution of international students executive summary*. Retrieved from http://www.acpet.edu.au/uploads/files/Reports_Submissions/213/Economic-Contribution-Executive-Summary.pdf

Baas, M. (2014). Victims or profiteers? Issues of migration, racism and violence among Indian students in Melbourne. *Asia Pacific Viewpoint, 55*(2), 212–225.

Biswas, R. R. (2014). Reverse migrant entrepreneurs in India: Motivations, trajectories and realities. In G. Tejada, U. Bhattacharya, B. Khadria, C. Kuptsch (Eds.), *Indian skilled migration and development: To Europe and back* (pp. 285–307). New Delhi: Springer.

Cemalcilar, Z., Falbo, T., & Stapleton, L. M. (2005). Cyber communication: A new opportunity for international students' adaptation? *International Journal of Intercultural Relations, 29*(1), 91–110.

Chib, A., Wilkin, H. A., & Hua, S. R. M. (2013). International migrant workers' use of mobile phones to seek social support in Singapore. *Information Technologies & International Development, 9*(4), 19–34.

Chib, A., Malik, S., Aricat, R. G., & Kadir, S. Z. (2014). Migrant mothering and mobile phones: Negotiations of transnational identity. *Mobile Media & Communication, 2*(1), 73–93.

Clark, N. (2013). *Vietnam: Trends in international and domestic education*. World Education News & Reviews. Retrieved from http://wenr.wes.org/213/06/vietnam-trends-in-international-and-domestic-education/

Constantine, M. G., Kindaichi, M., Okazaki, S., Gainor, K. A., & Baden, A. L. (2005). A qualitative investigation of the cultural adjustment experiences of Asian international college women. *Cultural Diversity and Ethnic Minority Psychology, 11*(2), 162.

Gupta, T. D., Man, G., Mirchandani, K., & Ng, R. (2014). Class Borders: Chinese and South Asian Canadian professional women navigating the labor market. *Asian and Pacific Migration Journal, 23*(1), 55.

Hirsch, E. (1992). The long term and the short term of domestic consumption. In R. Silverstone & E. Hirsch (Eds.), *Consuming technologies: Media and information in domestic spaces* (pp. 195–210). London: Routledge. Retrieved from the Taylor & Francis e-Library.

Hjorth, L. (2007). Home and away: A case study of the use of Cyworld mini-Hompy by Korean students studying in Australia. *Asian Studies Review, 31*(4), 397–407.

Hondagneu-Sotelo, P., & Avila, E. (1997). "I'm here, but I'm there" the meanings of Latina transnational motherhood. *Gender & Society, 11*(5), 548–571.

Kline, S. L., & Liu, F. (2005). The influence of comparative media use on acculturation, acculturative stress, and family relationships of Chinese international students. *International Journal of Intercultural Relations, 29*(4), 367–390.

Lang, X., Oreglia, E., & Thomas, S. (2010, September). Social practices and mobile phone use of young migrant workers. In *Proceedings of the 12th international conference on human computer interaction with mobile devices and services*, (pp. 59–62). New York: ACM.

Lee, J. W. Y., Kim, B., Lee, T. K., & Kim, M. S. (2012). Uncovering the use of facebook during an exchange program. *China Media Research, 8*(4), 62–76.

Lemor, A. M. R. (2006). Making a 'home'. The domestication of information and communication technologies in single parents' households. In T. Berker, M. Hartmann, Y. Punie, & K. J. Ward (Eds.), *Domestication of media and technology* (pp. 165–184). UK: McGraw-Hill Education.

Lie, M., & Sørensen, K. H. (2002). *Making technology of our own? Domesticating technology into everyday life* (pp. 1–30). Oslo: Scandinavian University Press.

Lim, S. S. (2008). Technology domestication in the Asian homestead: Comparing the experiences of middle class families in China and South Korea. *East Asian Science, Technology and Society, 2*(2), 189–209.

Lim, K., & Meier, E. B. (2012). International students' use of social network services in the new culture: A case study with Korean youths in the United States. *Asia Pacific Education Review, 13*(1), 113–120.

Madianou, M. (2012). Migration and the accentuated ambivalence of motherhood: The role of ICTs in Filipino transnational families. *Global Networks, 12*(3), 277–295.

Madianou, M., & Miller, D. (2011). Mobile phone parenting: Reconfiguring relationships between Filipina migrant mothers and their left-behind children. *New Media & Society, 13*(3), 457–470.

Mazzarol, T., & Soutar, G. N. (2002). "Push-pull" factors influencing international student destination choice. *International Journal of Educational Management, 16*(2), 82–90.

NAFSA. (2013). *The international student economic value tool*. Retrieved from http://www.nafsa.org/Explore_International_Education/Impact/Data_And_Statistics/The_International_Student_Economic_Value_Tool/

Romero, N., Markopoulos, P., Van Baren, J., De Ruyter, B., Ijsselsteijn, W., & Farshchian, B. (2007). Connecting the family with awareness systems. *Personal and Ubiquitous Computing, 11*(4), 299–312.

Sidhu, R. K. (2011). Re-thinking student migration trends, trajectories and rights. *National University of Singapore's Asia Research Institute*. Retrieved from http://www.ari.nus.edu.sg/docs/wps/wps11_157.pdf

Silverstone, R., Hirsch, E., & Morley, D. (1992). Information and communication technologies and the moral economy of the household. In R. Silverstone, & E. Hirsch (Eds.), *Consuming technologies: Media and information in domestic spaces* (pp. 12–28). London: Routledge. Retrieved from the Taylor & Francis e-Library.

Thomas, M., & Lim, S. S. (2011). On maids and mobile phones: ICT use by female migrant workers in Singapore and its policy implications. In J. E. Katz (Eds.), *Mobile communication: Dimensions of social policy* (pp. 175–190). New Brunswick: Transaction Publishers.

UNESCO Institute of Statistics. (2014). *Global flow of tertiary-level students*. Retrieved from http://www.uis.unesco.org/Education/Pages/international-student-flow-viz.aspx

Uy-Tioco, C. (2007). Overseas Filipino workers and text messaging: Reinventing transnational mothering. *Continuum: Journal of Media & Cultural Studies, 21*(2), 253–265.

Wood, N., & King, R. (2002). Media and migration: An overview. In N. Wood & R. King, (Eds.), *Media and migration: Constructions of mobility and difference* (pp. 1–22). London: Routledge

World Bank. (2013). *Migration and remittances*. Retrieved from http://web.worldbank.org/WBSITE/EXTERNAL/NEWS/0,,contentMDK:20648762~pagePK:64257043~piPK:437376~theSitePK:4607,00.html

Wyche, S. P., & Grinter, R. E. (2012). This is how we do it in my country: A study of computer-mediated family communication among Kenyan migrants in the united states. *Proceedings of the ACM 212 conference on Computer Supported Cooperative Work*, New York, pp. 87–96.

Yeoh, B., & Lin, W. (2012). Rapid growth in Singapore's immigration population brings policy challenges. *Migration Policy Institute*. Retrieved from http://www.migrationinformation.org/feature/display.cfm?ID=887

Part III
Strategies

Chapter 8
Restricting, Distracting, and Reasoning: Parental Mediation of Young Children's Use of Mobile Communication Technology in Indonesia

Laras Sekarasih

Abstract Using qualitative interviews for data-gathering, this study investigated how parents with young children (aged 2–7) in Indonesia's greater Jakarta area mediated their children's use of mobile communication devices. Parents introduce their children to smartphones or tablets for educational, entertainment, as well as "babysitting" purposes. However, parents' perceptions about online risks seem to outweigh those of benefits. Potential health issues, such as eyestrain and sedentary lifestyles, and exposure to violent content were seen as the most salient risks. Restrictive mediation on time and content was the most prevalent approach practiced, perhaps due to the age of the children and the lack of time and energy among working parents. In reaction to the children's resistance to time restrictions, parents with older children attempted to reason with the children and engage in parent–child conversations, while those with younger children preferred to redirect them to other activities.

Keywords Parental mediation • Restrictive mediation • Mobile communication • Digital technology • Online risks

Introduction

Mobile communication technologies increasingly provide opportunities for children to have their first interactions with information and communication technologies (ICTs). Recent data suggests that the penetration rate of mobile devices among families with children aged 8 and below was as high as 50 % in the EU countries (Holloway et al. 2013) and approximately 75 % in the United States (Common Sense Media 2013). The immediacy and interactivity of mobile

L. Sekarasih (✉)
University of Massachusetts, Amherst, MA, USA
e-mail: laras@issr.umass.edu

technology, as well as the simple interfaces of tablets and smartphones – relative to desktop computers and laptops – enable children to operate the devices with minimal assistance from adults (Holloway et al. 2013; Valkenburg 2004). On the one hand, mobile technology provides opportunities from which children can benefit (e.g., enhancing literacy and comfort with technology), yet on the other hand, it also poses online risks (e.g., violent and sexual content, online advertising, and disclosure of private information) which raise concerns among parents of young children (e.g., Donnerstein 2014; Livingstone 2011).

From the ecological perspective of human development, parents have direct influence over children's use of media and technology (Takeuchi and Levine 2014). Parents introduce children to different media forms and content, accompany and interact with them during "media time," as well as set boundaries around children's media consumption, in other words, exercising "parental mediation." In guiding children's media use, parents play a critical role in cultivating healthy and safe media habits as well as mitigating the undesirable influences of certain media (Clark 2011). The practice of parental mediation peaks in early childhood and wanes as the children enter adolescence (Livingstone and Helsper 2008; Nikken and Jansz 2014; Sonck et al. 2013; see also Warren 2003). However, existing studies on parental mediation of children's digital media use tend to focus on families with school-aged children and adolescents and less on those with very young children or toddlers (Clark 2011; Nikken and Jansz 2014). The present study aims to fill the gap in previous literature by investigating how parents, with children aged 2–7, guide and regulate young children's use of mobile communication technology.

The internet remains an emerging technology in Indonesia, the largest country in Southeast Asia and the fourth most populated country in the world. Currently, only 23 % of Indonesians are connected to the internet, due in part to the country's modest gross domestic product (GDP) as well as the technical challenge of building ICT infrastructure evenly throughout the archipelago (Christianto 2014; Pew Research Center 2014). At the same time, among Asia-Pacific's emerging economies, Indonesia was reported to be one of the fastest growing internet markets (Ling and Horst 2011; Telecompaper 2014). The adoption of mobile communication in Indonesia has also started to develop momentum: approximately 65 % of Indonesia's internet users go online using their smartphones or feature phones (Indonesia Association of Internet Service Providers 2013; The Nielsen Company 2011).

Relative to individuals in other parts of the country, residents of the Greater Jakarta area enjoy the privileges of better ICT infrastructure and higher GDP (Hill and Sen 2005; Statistics Indonesia 2012), which arguably facilitate the adoption of mobile communication technology. Although there is no data on the penetration rate of mobile devices among Indonesian families, it was reported that children in the cities spent more time using the internet than their parents, indicating the importance of mobile communication among Indonesia's young media users (Indonesia Association of Internet Service Providers 2013). Situated in the context of the Greater Jakarta area, Indonesia, this study examined how parents with young children aged 2–7 mediated their children's use of mobile communication technology.

Literature Review

Online Opportunities and Risks for Young Children

The internet creates various opportunities for young children to develop academic and social skills, as well as creativity and digital citizenship (see Holloway et al. (2013) for a review). Furthermore, in the contemporary context of kinship, where it is common for nuclear families to live far away from their extended families, the internet may also facilitate children's interaction and communication with their relatives (Ames et al. 2010). However, while using the internet may provide many potential benefits, it can also be risky for young children, especially considering their cognitive and emotional development. In a review on young children's responses to television programs, Valkenburg (2004) noted that 3-year-old children were still likely to approach television screens to wave or touch the characters they saw on it, which suggests children's difficulties in distinguishing between real life and 'reel' life. Drawing from Valkenburg's observation, one may argue that touchscreens' interactivity and immediate feedback might complicate children's ability to comprehend the imaginary or unrealistic aspects of media. Around age 5, children, especially boys, also begin to lose interest in educational content and become more attracted to programs that contain thrills or violence (Valkenburg 2004). In the context of mobile technology, this might raise the question of how long children will continue to be drawn to educational websites and applications.

Findings from previous research also suggest young children's vulnerability in comprehending the notion of online risks. For example, in a study on the perceptions of the internet among children aged 5–12, those in the 5- to 8-year-old age group showed limited understanding about the internet as a network, and minimal awareness about the potential positive and negative consequences of using the internet (Yan 2005). Ey and Cupit (2011) found that children aged 5–8 were able to identify some types of online risks (e.g., violence, obscenity, and interactions with strangers) but still showed susceptibility to scenarios that involved commercial messages, credibility of information, and disclosure of personal information. These previous studies probed into whether young children are cognitively and emotionally ready to fully benefit from ICTs as well as engage in safe and responsible online activities. The present study aimed to explore the issue from the parents' perspective by asking:

RQ1 How do parents weigh the possible benefits and harms of mobile technology for their young children?

Mediating Children's Use of the New Media

The existing body of literature on the use of television and video games in the family has documented three parental mediation strategies: active mediation, restrictive mediation, and co-viewing or co-using (e.g., Nathanson 2001; Nikken and Jansz

2006; Warren 2003). Active mediation refers to parent–child conversations about media in general and/or particular shows or games. Restrictive mediation is exercised by banning the use of certain media forms or content or imposing time limits on television viewing or video game playing. Finally, co-viewing/co-using takes place when parent and child watch television or play video games together. It is important to distinguish co-viewing/co-using from active mediation as the former does not necessarily involve parent–child dialogues.

The emergence of ICTs has prompted scholars to re-examine the applicability of the three aforementioned mediation strategies for children's television viewing in the context of new media. Livingstone and Helsper (2008) expanded the three types of parental mediation of television into four internet mediation approaches: *active co-use* (constructing parent–child conversations about the content of the internet and/or house rules on children's internet use while surfing the websites together), *interaction restriction* (limiting children's access to peer-to-peer interaction), *technical restriction* (installing filters or monitoring software), and *monitoring* (checking children's online activities such as looking at the browsing history after they finish using the internet). Sonck and colleagues (2013) attempted to replicate what Livingstone and Helsper found. However, their data from nationally representative Dutch families revealed slightly different types of internet mediation: *monitoring* (tracking children's e-mails, social network accounts, and previously visited websites), *restrictive content mediation* (setting rules and boundaries on what children can and cannot do online), *active safety mediation* (talking to children about online safety), and *restrictive technical mediation* (installing antivirus and website filters or setting timers to limit the time children spend online).

Arguing for the importance of investigating internet mediation among families with young children, Nikken and Jansz (2014) explored how parents guide their young children's internet use. In their nationally representative sample of Dutch parents with children aged 2–12 years old, the researchers found five commonly practiced mediation strategies. In *active mediation*, parents talk to children about responsible internet behaviors, including what to do about online strangers, protecting personal information, and cyberbullying. Parents can also *co-use* the internet with children. That is, at the parents' or children's initiative, parents and children surf the virtual world together or talk about the enjoyable aspects of the internet. *General restrictive mediation* refers to parental rules on whether children are allowed to play online games, which games they can play, and how long they can use the internet for. Somewhat similarly, in *content-specific restrictive mediation*, parents set the limit on what specific films, music, avatars, or consumer products children can see, listen to, use, or buy. Finally, parents exercise *supervision* by watching their children closely when they go online or only permit their children to surf the internet when parents are around.

It remains unclear whether parental mediation is effective in enhancing children's online experience and reducing online risks. Studies on the efficacy or perceived effectiveness of internet mediation have yielded mixed results. For example, Lee (2013) reported a negative correlation between limiting internet access and the amount of time children spend online in South Korean families with fourth- to ninth-grade children (see also Lee and Chae 2007). The researchers also found that restrictive mediation was associated with lower likelihood of exposure to online risks but did not negatively predict the likelihood of addictive internet use. In a qualitative study on parental socialisation of children's internet use among Singaporean parents with children aged 7–12, Shin (2013) found that among parents, the perceived benefits of the internet outweighed the perceived potential harms. Nevertheless, restrictive mediation, and not active mediation or co-using, came up as the most common mediation practice among the participants. For instance, children could only access the internet from shared computers that were located in the common area in the house and were also required to obtain parents' permission before going online. Shin also reported that parents expressed confidence in the effectiveness of restrictive mediation, which explained their preference for this approach in managing children's internet use (see also Nathanson et al. 2002; Padilla-Walker and Thompson 2005; Plowman et al. 2012).

In contrast, Livingstone and Helsper (2008) reported active co-use as the most commonly practiced approach among parents in their sample (i.e., UK parents with children aged 12–17). However, parental mediation was not associated with lower likelihood of children's engagement in risky online behaviors (e.g., accessing violent or pornographic content, interacting with strangers, and disclosing private information). Similarly, longitudinal data from a nationally representative sample of Flanders' fourth- to sixth-grade students suggest the ineffectiveness of internet mediation in reducing unsafe online behaviors (Valcke et al. 2011).

Previous studies have laid the basis for parental mediation research in the digital age by exploring the presence of different approaches of mediation strategies and, to some extent, tested the effectiveness of the practice. However, they might not be completely applicable for families with young children since they tend to focus on older children and adolescents, although many children today are exposed to digital media by the age of six (Calvert et al. 2005). Based on the existing literature, this study attempts to illuminate how parents manage their young children's use of mobile communication technology by asking:

RQ2 How do parents mediate their children's use of mobile technology? What strategies are used in their parental mediation practice?

Challenges in Mediating Children's Internet and Mobile Technology Use

Today's increasing use of mobile technology has also challenged and complicated the practice of parental mediation. Jiow and Lim (2012) charted the affordances of newer generation video games and their implications for parental mediation, which can inform our understanding of the mobile communication landscape. They argue that the portability of mobile devices exerts challenges for parents to exercise close observation and supervision, since looking at the small screens of computers, tablets, or cell phones together is impractical and inconvenient (see also Livingstone and Helsper 2008). As well, the convergence of media platforms has enabled children to access mobile applications (hereafter, apps) and online content from multiple forms and channels. Consequently, parents now have to monitor all accessible platforms and devices in order to track and manage their children's mobile technology use. In addition to the features of mobile media itself, the general technical aspects of the internet also pose challenges for parents, especially those who are less savvy or lack the confidence to interact with technology (Livingstone and Helsper 2008; Nikken and Jansz 2014). The issue of familiarity and comfort in using the internet and mobile technology also challenges traditional gender-based roles among parents (Livingstone 2011). Mothers traditionally assume the responsibility of managing children's media use, while fathers are responsible for technology-related issues. However, the ubiquity of mobile media necessitates that families revisit such parental "division of labor," which adds another layer of complexity to parental mediation practice. Hence, the current study also aims to explore the challenges that parents face in mediating their young children's mobile technology use by asking:

RQ3 What challenges do parents face in managing their young children's use of mobile communication technology?

Method

This study employs a qualitative approach, using semi-structured interviews as a data-collection method. Interview questions were constructed based on existing literature on parental mediation and ICT infrastructure in Jakarta. Twenty-three interviews (with 21 mothers and 2 fathers) were conducted in June and July 2014. Participants were recruited through convenience sampling by reaching out to the researcher's network of friends and acquaintances. At the time of the interviews, all participants had at least one child who was between the ages of 2 and 7 (three participants had more than one child whose ages fell within the 2–7 age range) and resided in the Greater Jakarta metropolitan area (i.e., Jakarta and its surrounding satellite areas, such as Bekasi and Tangerang). The predominantly maternal sample was consistent with many existing parental mediation studies, where mothers constituted the majority of participants in the studies (see, e.g., Nikken and Jansz 2014; Warren 2003).

Participants' ages ranged between 29 and 36 years. 18 out of the 23 participants held a full-time job – only two mothers worked part time and three were full-time parents. Most participants were college educated (one held a 3-year vocational diploma and seven held a graduate degree), and all were from middle- to upper-middle-class socioeconomic backgrounds. The sample was appropriate for the purpose of the study, as they possess the economic resources to own mobile communication devices and the fact that they all resided in the Greater Jakarta area, where Indonesia's ICT infrastructure is concentrated (Hills and Sen 2005). All participants had more than one mobile device available in their households (at least one smartphone for each of them and their spouses). The summary of participants' demographic characteristics is available in the Appendix.

The proposal for this study was approved by the departmental human subject review. Due to the participants' work schedule, only five interviews were conducted in person, and the remaining 18 were conducted by phone. All interviews were conducted in the national language, Indonesia (also known as *Bahasa Indonesia*). The duration of the interviews ranged between 18 and 50 minutes, averaging 35 minutes. Oral consent was obtained at the beginning of each interview. Participants were informed about the broad purpose of the study (i.e., studying the use of electronic media, including handheld gadgets, in the family), length of the interviews, and confidentiality. They were also assured that there were no wrong or right answers, and they retained the right to skip any interview questions as well as to leave the study at any point. All interviews were recorded with the participants' consent and transcribed in Indonesian. The length of the transcripts ranged between 868 and 4700 words.

Participants' responses were then analyzed by the researcher with the assistance of NVivo 10 software. Emerging themes were identified using constant comparison methods (Charmaz 2006; Lindlof and Taylor 2002). Coding was initially performed by running a word frequency count in NVivo in order to explore the broad themes that emerged. When a "keyword" that frequently appeared was found (e.g., "time," "limit"), the context of the sentences in which the word came up was checked to identify a tentative theme. Once a theme was tentatively established, related keywords and sentences were compared to determine whether they formed a new theme or could be merged with the existing themes. This process was repeated until the saturation point was reached. Once emerging themes were confirmed by additional examples, representative exemplars were selected to illustrate the trends. All names of parents and children that appeared in the findings are pseudonyms and the presented exemplars are English translations of the Indonesian interview transcripts.

Findings

Parents' Perceptions about Potential Benefits and Harms of Mobile Technology

Most participants reported that they introduced their children to mobile communication technology, such as smartphones or tablets, within the children's first 5 years, with the intention of teaching them alphabets, numbers, children's songs, or English words. Irma (32), the mother of Oscar (4), said that she purchased an iPad and installed educational apps for Oscar when he was a year old. She shared that Oscar indeed benefited from the apps: "Like reciting ABC, A to Z, he learned it by himself. [Also] numbers and counting… he learned them on his own."

Mobile devices were also used to encourage the children to remain seated during mealtimes or during family trips, as well as to provide them with alternatives to watching television. Citing the lack of safety in the area where his family lived, Aryo (34), one of the two fathers in the study, explained that he actually preferred that his daughter play with the iPad instead of outdoors with her peers in the neighborhood. Additionally, some parents believed that involving technology in today's family life was inevitable. Rico (36), another father in this study said, "Gadgets are part of today's daily life, so I don't have any problem introducing them to my kids."

While participants reported the positive aspects of mobile devices for their young children, concerns about the problematic aspects of the technology seemed to be more salient than its perceived benefits. Two mothers even declared that introducing their children to the iPad was "a mistake." Parents associated mobile technology with health- and behavior-related issues, such as eyestrain, sleep deprivation, a sedentary lifestyle, and internet addiction. Some participants mentioned that gadgets would reduce their children's interest to engage in outdoor and physical activities and compromise on the development of their interpersonal skills. The portability of tablets or smartphones, which enabled them to bring the gadgets to bed, was also noted as interfering with the children's sleep schedules.

However, concerns about health-related issues seemed to be secondary to the anxiety about objectionable online or mobile app content. Exposure to obscenity and media violence emerged most frequently among participants. For some parents, children were more likely to encounter objectionable content on mobile devices than on television. Unlike watching videos on YouTube, television viewing could actually be safer for kids, since there were television channels – especially on cable – whose programs were specifically designed for children. Hanifah (34), whose iPad was mostly loaded with children's games applications (e.g., jigsaws, music instruments, cake decorating games) and cartoon movies (e.g., Disney's *Frozen*), restricted her daughters from browsing clips on YouTube. She even decided to uninstall YouTube from the iPad in order to eliminate the possibility of her eldest daughter Mia (5), who was already able to spell and type simple and familiar words, accidentally finding pornographic clips:

> She already knows how to write "Princess". She might start by searching "Princess" videos … [but] there are always clips in the list of suggested videos that are not related to what she is looking for…[including] those "weird" [pornographic] clips.

Besides exposure to sexual images, parents were also worried that their children would reproduce physical or verbal aggressions they were exposed to through games or online videos. Tisha (30), a mother of two, was appalled when she once checked the YouTube search history on her iPad and found a clip that contained profanity. She presumed that her son Raymond (5) had unintentionally accessed the video: "It must have appeared among the list of 'related videos'." Not wanting Raymond to imitate the foul language, Tisha deleted the video from the iPad's history and told Raymond's nanny to supervise the boy's iPad use more closely.

Likewise, Medina (35) felt troubled with the *Batman* games that her son Zaki (5) played on the iPad. According to Medina, it was Zaki's father – her husband – who chose and installed the games for the boy. Unfortunately, not only did Zaki enjoy playing them, he also started to imitate the fighting scenes he saw in the games. Medina said, "Of course [he imitates it]! Pow! Kapow! (imitating the fight words). He bounces around. His little brother will get hurt if he at some point becomes Zaki's punch bag." However, Medina did not remove the games from the iPad, partly because her son already had an affinity for superheroes like *Batman* and *Captain America*. Raihana (33), another participant, was also concerned about her son Reza's (4) attraction to characters from *The Avengers*, yet she noted that "it's impossible to completely ban superheroes from boys."

Three parents brought up the fear of having dangerous online interaction with strangers. Ratri (30), for example, did not allow her daughter Davina (2) to play with her and her husband's smartphones at all except for retrieving photos and videos from the phones' internal memory. She or her husband also always stayed near Davina whenever the girl was playing with the phones. In addition to feeling worried about internet addiction and sedentary lifestyle, Ratri said that she wanted to prevent the risk of contact with online sexual predators. As a lawyer, she had heard about criminal cases that involved pictures of children that were downloaded from social media: "[Children] don't realise that [their] pictures can get into the wrong hands. I heard from my colleagues about children's pictures that circulate among pedophiles…[Those images] must be obtained from social media."

Likewise, Anggita (32) stood by her decision to heavily limit her son Adrian's (3) use of the iPad. She recognised that this would possibly undermine the development of his technological knowledge and skills, but she believed that the stringent restriction would be worth the delay. Anggita said that she wanted to buy some time to equip Adrian with the knowledge of online risks, especially pertaining to dangerous encounters with strangers.

Only two mothers – Medina and Mirna – mentioned objections to online advertising. Medina disliked *EvanTubeHD*, a YouTube channel that reviews various children's toys such as *Star Wars* action figures or *Play-Doh*, because "Zaki always nags for toys that he sees in the videos." Somewhat similarly, based on past experience with television advertisements, which made her daughter Alicia (5) ask for unhealthy food products that had been advertised, Mirna (32) told Alicia to skip the commercials that preceded some popular clips on YouTube.

In sum, the perceived risks of using mobile devices seemed to outweigh the benefits. The potential benefits of using smartphones and tablets were perceived as being easily replaceable by other (traditional) media. Some parents even argued that they preferred paper books, pencils or crayons, jigsaw puzzles, and board games to teach their children letters, numbers, or shapes over facilitating their children's learning with educational mobile apps. Traditional, nonelectronic media were seen as safer, more stimulating, and useful for motor skill development and social interactions. In contrast, participants perceived that mobile communication technology created risks that were worse than the negative influences of other electronic media such as television.

Restrictive Mediation as the Primary Mediation Strategy

Time Restriction

Restrictive mediation (both time and content) emerged as the most frequently cited parental mediation strategy among participants. Parents reported that they set limits and rules in order to prevent their children from viewing problematic content or developing unhealthy media habits. Working parents delegated this task to other caregivers (e.g., extended family members or nannies) when they were not at home. Almost all parents mentioned time restriction as part of their mediation strategy. The time limit that was imposed on children varied from 15 minutes to 4 hours a day, and some parents only allowed their children to use handheld gadgets on weekends. Referring to the clock (e.g., "You can play until the long hand points toward number 6.") and days (e.g., "Today is Thursday. You can play with iPad on Saturday.") and deciding how many more rounds of games or YouTube clips the kids could play or watch (e.g., "Two more clips, and then we go to bed.") were the commonly used strategies to signal time limit.

Parents' responses suggest that the decisions to curb the amount of time their children could spend with mobile devices were motivated by the intention to minimise the potential detriments of handheld gadgets to children's health and social skills. Intan (30), a mother in the study, no longer lets her son Daniel (3) play with the iPad because he became inactive and was on the gadget all day. Likewise, Astri (32) said that she limited her son Abian's (2) touchscreen time to 2 hours per day. She would rather Abian "play something outdoors, like football" because "playing with tablet lacks [the element of] social interaction."

Content Restriction

Parental concerns about exposure to sex and violence seemed to prompt them to set boundaries on what their children could access. Children were told not to watch or play certain videos and games, respectively, and had to seek permission to download game apps. Hanifah (34), who uninstalled YouTube from her iPad, repeatedly expressed her deep concern about the possibility of her daughter Mia (5) seeing sexual images on YouTube. She preloaded Mia's favorite videos on the device, so that the latter would not need to browse YouTube to look for clips. Knowing Mia's fear of horror movies, Hanifah deliberately misled her daughter about the existence of horror videos on YouTube. She realised that lying to Mia was not a good parenting practice, but decided to tell such stories anyway, because she was not ready to answer questions about sexual images:

> If I don't scare her….I don't know what else I can do. Scaring my child is not the best thing to do… I feel bad for her. But if I allow her [watch YouTube clips], I'm really worried that she would accidentally see that weird stuff. Once she saw those scenes, I know she would

be curious and ask me questions. That's why I scare her with stories about clips from horror movies.

Hanifah was the only parent who went as far as to uninstall YouTube from her iPad, but she was not alone in her discomfort with sexual content. In fact, many parents in this study did not even say the word "sexual," "pornographic," or "suggestive" in their responses. Instead, they used euphemisms like "weird images" or "not-for-children content."

Restrictive mediation was often exercised in conjunction with other parental mediation techniques, especially technical restriction and supervision/monitoring. Most participants said that they placed themselves near their children when the latter were playing with gadgets in order to keep track of the time and to ensure that no objectionable content was accessed and felt confident that their children would only see age-appropriate content if supervision was in place. In other words, supervision was an avenue for parents to enforce time and content restriction. Rana (31) reported that her daughter Andhari (2) never played with gadgets by herself. Rana always made sure that a caregiver – herself, her husband, or the nanny – was nearby when Andhari was using the tablet. Additionally, she also created a separate YouTube account for her daughter, enabled the application's *Safety Mode* feature, and checked the account's browsing history in order to make sure that Andhari did not watch clips that contained violence or sex.

Addressing Children's Resistance to Parental Mediation

In general, parents in this study reported that their children were relatively compliant with the content restrictions that they impose. However, when it came to time restriction, many complained that their children had started to resist the house policies that limit their time to play with gadgets. Notably, the way the children expressed their resistance seemed to vary depending on their age. In general, parents with toddlers (roughly between 2 and 4 years old) reported that their children whined, screamed, or cried to express their discontentment when the smartphones or tablets were taken away. In contrast, older children (5 years or older) resisted by arguing or talking back to their parents. The age-based variation in children's assertiveness and ability to articulate their wants and opinions reflected the difference in their cognitive and linguistic development.

Consequently, parents' strategies in addressing the resistance varied accordingly as well. Parents with toddlers said that they usually redirected the children to other toys or activities. According to them, trying to talk to the children would only incite more crying or tantrums. Due to toddlers' shorter attention spans, once parents managed to divert them from smartphones or tablets, the children would be preoccupied with the new activities and "forget" about the gadgets. Astri (32), for example, would start a hide-and-seek game using pillows and blankets in the bedroom to stop her son playing with her tablet.

In contrast, parents with older children (aged 5–7) responded to their children's resistance by reasoning with them about the necessity of time limits. Nanda (34), for instance, who only allowed her son Alam (7) to play with her tablet before she went to work and on weekends, reminded him that the tablet was primarily purchased for work purposes:

> He has no choice in the morning when I take away the tablet for work. [I say,] "I'm leaving for work, I need the tablet." [He says,] "Why can't you just leave it with me?" [I say,] "No. I need it to communicate with my colleagues. ... Remember that I bought this tablet for work."

Nanda also explained to Alam the possible health problems associated with excessive gadget use, for example, eyestrain. This explanation, however, did not always work, as he was ready with replies like "I can go to the doctor to cure the eyestrain." Citra (32), the mother of Lea (5) and Laksmi (3), used both strategies of distraction and dialogue. She told the girls that too much playing with tablets and smartphones would cause learning difficulties and reminded the girls how much the devices had caused quarrels between them. At the same time, admitting Laksmi's persistence in asking to play with gadgets, Citra also hid her smartphone and tablet at home as much as possible and persuaded the children to play with toys like *Lego*.

The unreliable internet connection surprisingly served as an opportunity for parents to make their children stop playing with the handheld devices, especially watching YouTube videos, which required good data connection for streaming. Recounting her constant struggle in making her daughter Adeline (2) quit playing with her iPhone, Lana (31) said, "I'm actually glad when the connection is lagging, because I can tell her, 'Look, the internet is not working. Let's play something else'." Likewise, Ajeng said that slow connections had a "bright side," because when a YouTube clip buffered for too long, her son Ken (3) would leave the iPad to play with other toys. Again, toddlers' short attention spans prompted them to quickly shift from playing with gadgets to doing other activities.

Similarly, Mirna (32) used a bad signal reception as a way to keep Alicia (5) away from her iPhone. However, unlike Lana and Ajeng, whose children would instantly move on to playing with other toys, Mirna had to reason and "prove" to the girl the presence of the technical issue:

> [I say,] "See…there's no reception." [She says,] "Yes, there is. It says '3G', not 'E'." [I say,] "Why don't you try it?" She has to see it herself that we don't have data reception. If it takes too long for a video to load, she eventually will say, "I'll play with something else."

In sum, families differed in the way they addressed children's resistance to time limits on their mobile device use based on the children's age. Families with older children might engage in dialogues about the possible harms of handheld gadgets in response to the children's resistance to parents' restrictive mediation. In contrast, parents with toddlers tended to deploy alternative activities or toys as a solution.

Resistance and Support from Family Members

The dynamics among immediate and extended family members in managing the use of mobile technology also emerged in participants' responses. Most mothers in the study said that they assumed more authority than their husbands in regulating the children's screen time; however, some said that they and their spouses were not always a united front in mediating their children's use of mobile devices. Lamenting their husbands' inconsistencies or leniency, they also figured that their children preferred playing with their fathers' phones not only because the device had more interesting games but also because fathers were more relaxed about letting the children use them. Besides feeling frustrated, mothers were also afraid that the children would get confused about the house rules or inadvertently identify the parents as "good cop" and "bad cop." Alina (29), for example, said that her husband Farhan was an avid smartphone user and was relatively relaxed about how much their daughter Airin (3) could use his smartphone. Airin was not allowed to play with Alina's phone, but Farhan often let the girl play with his. Alina said:

> There was this "episode" in our family…when her father came home, Airin was instantly on her feet and asked him for his cell phone. Once she played with it, she refused to let go, even when my husband needed the phone to send business e-mails…. He was upset about it. I said to him, "If you don't want Airin to play with your phone, then you yourself should not be constantly on the phone."

Challenges in creating a consistent mediation practice could also come from the extended family. Grandparents, aunts, or uncles tended to accommodate children's requests, which made it difficult to enforce rules and boundaries that participants set as parents. Lila (34), whose parents helped watch her son Anggara (4), lamented that enforcing the 2-hour screen time was challenging, partly because her parents – Anggara's grandparents – were permissive. Lila said:

> His grandparents let him play with the smartphones almost as much as he wants…. Anggara always asks for my permission if he wants to play with my phone…[but] with my mom's phone…he just grabs it, enters the passcode, and plays the games on it.

Lila and some other mothers who struggled to foster consistency in regulating their children's screen time were able to partially solve this problem by asking the members of the extended families to comply with their parental authority and help them enforce the rules on their children's media use. However, for some others, dealing with relatives was a delicate matter. Raihana (33), for example, had to tread the fine line between limiting her son's smartphone use and maintaining a good relationship with her in-laws. Raihana only allowed her son Reza (4) to play with her or her husband's phone for a total of half an hour per day. However, she found it almost impossible to implement the rule when Reza stayed over at her in-laws', because he "can play with his aunt's iPhone whenever he wants." Raihana decided not to confront her in-laws despite her frustration and instead tried to understand that their leniency with Reza for two reasons. First, until a few weeks prior to the interview, Reza was their only grandchild and nephew, and he did not get to see his grandparents and aunt regularly. Second, the in-laws' availability to babysit Reza on some weekends gave Raihana and her husband time to run errands without having to worry about their son.

Discussion

This study examined how parents of young children aged 2–7 managed their kids' use of mobile communication technology, such as smartphones or tablets, focusing on how parents weighed the possible benefits and harms of mobile technology for their young children, the parental mediation approaches they used, and challenges they encountered in mediation. Parents reported that they introduced their children to mobile devices for educational (e.g., teaching children alphabets and numbers), babysitting (e.g., keeping children sit still during mealtime), and entertainment-oriented purposes. However, parents' responses also revealed concerns regarding how mobile technology might lead to health-related issues (e.g., physically inactive lifestyle, internet addiction, eyestrain), exposure to problematic content (e.g., violence, sex, and advertising), and contact with strangers. Overall, parental concerns about the risks of using mobile communication devices seemed to outweigh the perceived benefits of the technology.

Restrictive mediation on time and content was the primary approach among parents in this study. Parents' preferences for setting boundaries on how long children could use tablets or smartphones and the kinds of applications they were allowed to access were consistent with previous parental mediation studies (e.g., Livingstone and Helsper 2008; Nikken and Jansz 2014; Shin 2013; Warren 2003). The prevalence of restrictive mediation can be attributed to three factors. First, the salience of potential risks of mobile technology, which was greater than that of perceived potential affordances, might have prompted parents to limit their children's access to the technology. Furthermore, restrictive mediation was also propelled by the anxiety about age-inappropriate images, especially those with sexual or violent content, and parents' lack of self-efficacy in discussing objectionable content with their children (Nathanson et al. 2002). Second, implementing rules is considerably more practical and realisable than engaging in parent–child dialogues about internet content and safety, especially for families with working parents (Warren 2003). Third, the preference for restrictive mediation is also attributable to young children's psychological development. Compared to active mediation, restrictive mediation requires less cognitive and emotional efforts from both parents and children. Since young children are still limited in their language and reasoning capability, restricting the amount of time and the types of content they can access might be more effective than reasoning with them. In this study, different approaches in handling children's resistance to screen time rules suggest parents' awareness of children's age as a factor to consider in guiding the use of mobile technology in the family. Parents with toddlers (around the age of 2–4) addressed their children's whines and nags – the way the kids expressed their anger when parents took away the gadgets – by diverting their children's attention toward other toys or activities. In contrast, those whose children were older (aged 5–7) – and were already able to argue with their parents – tried to engage in conversation about house rules, possible health risks, or technical issues of using handheld devices.

Besides having to manage children's reactance, parents also had to deal with resistance from their own spouses and relatives. Specifically, participants complained that the leniency of other family members compromised the effectiveness of the time restriction they tried to enforce. Some parents resolved this problem by asserting their authority as parents, but others decided not to voice their objection in order to maintain good relationships especially with their extended families. Future studies are needed to examine whether such dynamics among nuclear and extended family members differ across cultures.

This study has limitations that should be acknowledged. Parents in this study might not be free from social desirability on "what they thought they should do." Thus, the responses might not truly reflect what actually happens in the family (Sonck et al. 2013), but instead how the parents wish to portray of themselves. The portability of mobile devices and the fact that most parents in this study worked full time might have also made it challenging for participants to accurately recall their children media habits. Combined, those factors might have led parents to underreport their children's use of mobile technology, and/or overestimated the frequency, stringency, and effectiveness of their parental mediation practice. Future studies should include the perspectives of the children in order to fill this possible gap, as well as assess the effectiveness of the mediation strategies. The use of telephone interviews as a data-gathering method also posed some challenges, as it limited the researcher's ability to capture participants' nonverbal cues, as well as physical aspects of their home environment. However, since most participants in this study worked full time with schedules that did not enable the researcher to conduct face-to-face interviews, phone interviews were the only logistically feasible option to collect data.

In spite of its limitations, this study illuminates the practice of parental mediation of mobile communication technology among families with young children. It contributes to the body of literature on parental mediation, especially on the use of digital technology among families with young children, which has not been frequently investigated in previous research. Furthermore, this study also offers practical implications for designers to make devices and apps more family-friendly. For instance, designers can help parents exercise time restrictions and alleviate parental concerns about the health and behavioral issues associated with too much screen time by enabling a "time limit" feature on the device or app. Mobile apps designers might also want to make age-based content ratings more prominent to make it easier for parents to see and teach their children which apps are appropriate for them. Lastly, this study also offers insights for media education practitioners on the perceived opportunities and risks of mobile communication technology, which may prompt the development of educational initiatives that aim to cultivate safe and informed use of such devices in the family.

Appendix: Participants' Demographic Profiles

Demographic attributes	Younger children (aged 2 to 4)	Older children (aged 5 to 7)
Participants' (parents) gender		
Mothers	14	9
Fathers	1	1
Participants' age		
29–30	4	1
31–33	9	2
34–36	2	7
Participants' educational attainment		
Associate degree	1	0
College degree	8	8
Graduate degree	6	2
Children's gender		
Girls	9	7
Boys	8	3
Children's age		
2 years old	4	
3 years old	9	
4 years old	4	
5 years old		7
6 years old		2
7 years old		1
Devices that children frequently used		
iPhone	4	2
iPad	4	4
Android smartphone	4	1
Android tablet	2	4
(Not allowing child to play with devices at all)	2	0
Genres of frequently used applications		
Educational (e.g., *Sesame Street*, *Fisher Price's* applications)	12	5
Entertainment oriented (e.g., *Angry Birds*, *Batman*, salon game applications)	14	10
YouTube	15	10

The numbers do not add up to 23 (the number of participants in the study), because three participants had more than one children. Children might also have access to more than one type of gadget

References

Ames, M. G., Go, J., Kaye, J., & Spasojevic, M. (2010). Making love in the network closet: The benefits and work of family videochat. *Proceedings of the 2010 ACM Conference on Computer Supported Cooperative Work*, 145–154.

Calvert, S. L., Rideout, V. J., Woolard, J. L., Barr, R. F., & Strousse, G. A. (2005). Age, ethnicity, and socioeconomic patterns in early computer use: A national survey. *American Behavioral Scientist, 58*(7), 590–607.

Charmaz, K. (2006). *Constructing grounded theory: A practical guide through qualitative research*. London: Sage.

Christianto, I. (2014). IT & gadgets: Broadband available for all. http://www.thejakartapost.com/news/2014/04/08/it-gadgets-broadband-available-all.html. Accessed 27 May 2014,

Clark, L. S. (2011). Parental mediation theory for the digital age. *Communication Theory, 21*(4), 323–343.

Common Sense Media. (2013). *Zero to eight: Children's media use in America 2013*. https://www.commonsensemedia.org/research/zero-to-eight-childrens-media-use-in-america-2013. Accessed 30 Nov 2014.

Donnerstein, E. (2014). The internet. In V. C. Strasburger, B. J. Wilson, & A. B. Jordan (Eds.), *Children, adolescents, and the media* (3rd ed.), Thousand Oaks: Sage.

Ey, L., & Cupit, C. G. (2011). Exploring young children's understanding of risks associated with internet usage and their concepts of management strategies. *Journal of Early Childhood Research, 9*(1), 53–65.

Hill, D. T., & Sen, K. (2005). *The internet in Indonesia's new democracy*. Oxon: Routledge.

Holloway, D., Green, L., & Livingstone, S. (2013). *Zero to eight: Young children and their internet use*. LSE, London: EU Kids Online.

Indonesia Association of internet Service Provider (Asosiasi Jasa Penyelenggara internet Indonesia) (2013). *Indonesia internet user profile (profil pengguna internet indonesia) 2012*. Jakarta: APJII.

Jiow, H. J., & Lim, S. S. (2012). The evolution of video game affordances and implications for parental mediation. *Bulletin of Science, Technology & Society, 32*(6), 455–462.

Lee, S. (2013). Parental restrictive mediation of children's internet use: Effective for what and for whom? *New Media & Society, 15*(4), 466–481.

Lee, S., & Chae, Y. (2007). Children's internet use in a family context: Influence on family relationships and parental mediation. *CyberPsychology & Behavior, 10*(5), 640–644.

Lindlof, T. R., & Taylor, B. C. (2002). *Qualitative communication research methods* (2nd ed.). Thousand Oaks: Sage Publications.

Ling, R., & Horst, H. A. (2011). Mobile communication in the global south. *New Media & Society, 13*(3), 363–374.

Livingstone, S. (2011). Internet, children, and youth. In M. Consalvo & C. Ess (Eds.), *The handbook of internet studies* (pp. 348–368). Malden: Wiley-Blackwell.

Livingstone, S., & Helsper, E. J. (2008). Parental mediation of children's internet use. *Journal of Broadcasting & Electronic Media, 52*(4), 581–599.

Nathanson, A. I. (2001). Parent and child perspectives on the presence and meaning of parental television mediation. *Journal of Broadcasting & Electronic Media, 45*(2), 201–220.

Nathanson, A. I., Eveland Jr, W. P., Park, H., & Paul, B. (2002). Perceived media influence and efficacy as predictors of caregivers' protective behaviors. *Journal of Broadcasting & Electronic Media, 46*(3), 385–410.

Nikken, P., & Jansz, J. (2006). Parental mediation of children's videogame playing: A comparison of the reports by parents and children. *Learning, Media and Technology, 31*(2), 181–202.

Nikken, P., & Jansz, J. (2014). Developing scales to measure parental mediation of young children's internet use. *Learning, Media and Technology, 39*(2), 250–266.

Padilla-Walker, L. M., & Thompson, R. A. (2005). Combating conflicting messages of values: A closer look at parental strategies. *Social Development, 14*(2), 305–323.

Pew Research Center. (2014). Emerging nations embrace internet, mobile technology. http://www.pewglobal.org/files/2014/02/Pew-Research-Center-Global-Attitudes-Project-Technology-Report-FINAL-February-13-20146.pdf. Accessed 27 May 2014.

Plowman, L., Stevenson, O., Stephen, C., & McPake, J. (2012). Preschool children's learning with technology at home. *Computers & Education, 59*(1), 30–37.

Shin, W. (2013). Parental socialization of children's internet use: A qualitative approach. *New Media & Society.* Advance online publication. doi: 10.1177/1461444813516833.

Sonck, N., Nikken, P., & de Haan, J. (2013). Determinants of internet mediation: A comparison of the reports by Dutch parents and children. *Journal of Children and Media, 7*(1), 96–113.

Statistics Indonesia (Badan Pusat Statistik). (2012). Trends of selected socio-economic indicators of Indonesia. http://www.bps.go.id/booklet/Booklet_Agustus_2012.pdf. Accessed 27 May 2014.

Takeuchi, L., & Levine, M. (2014). Learning in a digital age: Toward a new ecology of human development. In A. B. Jordan & D. Romer (Eds.), *Media and the well-being of children and adolescents* (pp. 20–43). New York: Oxford University Press.

Telecompaper. (2014). *Fixed broadband connections to jump 5.7 % per year by end-2015.* http://www.telecompaper.com/news/fixed-broadband-connections-to-jump-57-per-yr-by-end-2015--1019247. Accessed 1 Dec 2014.

The Nielsen Company. (2011). The digital media habits and attitudes of southeast Asian consumers. http://www.nielsen.com/content/dam/corporate/us/en/reports-downloads/2011-Reports/South-East-Asia-Digital-Consumer.pdf. Accessed 27 May 2014.

Valcke, M., De Wever, B., Van Keer, H., & Schellens, T. (2011). Long-term study of safe internet use of young children. *Computers & Education, 57*(1), 1292–1305.

Valkenburg, P. M. (2004). *Children's responses to the screen: A media psychological approach.* Mahwah: Routledge.

Warren, R. (2003). Parental mediation of preschool children's television viewing. *Journal of Broadcasting & Electronic Media, 47*(3), 394–417.

Yan, Z. (2005). Age differences in children's understanding of the complexity of the internet. *Journal of Applied Developmental Psychology, 26*(4), 385–396.

Chapter 9
Paradoxes in the Mobile Parenting Experiences of Filipino Mothers in Diaspora

Ma. Rosel S. San Pascual

Abstract This chapter illuminates the paradoxes in the mobile parenting experiences of Filipino mothers in diaspora as it describes the attempts of these migrant mothers to parent their children in spite of their spatial and temporal separation. Three pairs of paradoxes were uncovered from the author's analysis of the interviews conducted among 32 Singapore-based Filipino working mothers about their mediated parenting experiences: the independence/dependence paradox, competence/incompetence paradox, and empowerment/enslavement paradox. The exposed paradoxes indicate that the mobile parenting experiences of these migrant mothers are not entirely celebratory as positive mediated experiences coexist with negative ones. And yet, for these migrant mothers, even though mobile parenting engenders paradoxes in mediated experiences, they nonetheless regard it as the best response to the situation imposed by their transnational separation.

Keywords Mobile parenting • Mediated parenting • Migrant mothers • Technology paradox • Transnational family

The Filipino Family in the Age of Diaspora

"Family" is both a social construct and a lived reality. As a socially constructed concept, our society presents us with normative prescriptions of what a family is and how a family should be. Parreñas (2005a) wrote that, "In any given society, people hold ideas about what families are supposed to be, what activities different members are supposed to do, how they are supposed to behave, and what immediate experiences members are supposed to gain from the routines and norms of family life" (p. 33). As a lived reality, each of us has experienced some form of family. Parreñas (2005a) remarked that the experience of family is "rooted in patterns of shared activities" among "men, women, and children who share material sources

---

M.R.S. San Pascual (✉)
University of the Philippines, Diliman, Quezon City, Philippines
e-mail: mssanpascual@up.edu.ph

© Springer Science+Business Media Dordrecht 2016
S.S. Lim (ed.), *Mobile Communication and the Family*, Mobile Communication in Asia: Local Insights, Global Implications,
DOI 10.1007/978-94-017-7441-3_9

and in cooperation and sometimes conflict provide one another with material, physical, and emotional care" (p. 33).

Filipinos place tremendous, unquestionable value on their family (Medina 2001). Even in light of the growth in the number of Filipinos leaving their home and country to pursue better economic and career opportunities overseas has given rise to increasing numbers of Filipino transnational families, maintaining strong family ties remains the foremost priority. Asis et al. (2004) observed that, "While transnational migration is reshaping the contours of the Filipino family, it has in no way diminished the importance of being, or the desire to be, "family"" (p. 204).

Filipinos work to maintain strong affective ties with their families. Opportunely, the rise in the number of transnational Filipino families has coincided with the emergence of innovative communication media and technologies. Thus, while the postmodern era broadened the permeability of national borders, which increased the fluidity of transnational mobility, it also ushered in advanced communication media and technologies, which have made long-distance communication more accessible and affordable to transnational family members. A growth in inexpensive options for overseas communication has made global interconnections more tenable (Aguilar et al. 2009; Paragas 2008; Vertovec 2004).

This chapter describes the attempts of Filipino migrant mothers to parent their children in spite of their geographical distance from them. This chapter also explores the dissonance in these mothers' mediated parenting experiences and their struggles as they persist in parenting their children even though society fundamentally treats transnational parenting as far from ideal.

Spatial and Temporal Factors in Communication and Parenting

Present-day communication media and technologies enable connections between and among transnational family members irrespective of geographical space and time. As Katz and Aakhus (2002) put it, contemporary forms of media and technologies allow migrant families to be in perpetual contact with one another. Without a doubt, "connection mobility complements global mobility" (San Pascual 2014b, p. 195).

Mobile phones revolutionised long-distance contact among transnational family members by increasing the potential for simultaneity (Paragas 2008). During the age of land-based phones, telephone calls had to be planned beforehand so that family members would be present to receive the prearranged overseas land-based call at the agreed upon time (Aguilar et al. 2009; Paragas 2005). Before the era of mobile communication, transnational family members were tied to a particular space and a specific time to be able to engage in long-distance communication. As Chu and Yang (2006) noted, "people have been brought into a new era where they can engage in communication that is free from the constraints of physical proximity and spatial immobility" (p. 223). This technological advancement has had significant effects on the transnational parenting practices of parents in diaspora (Madianou and Miller 2011, 2012a; 2012b; San Pascual 2014a, b; Uy-Tioco 2007).

Parenting refers to "purposive activities aimed at ensuring the survival and development of children" (Hoghughi 2004, p. 5). It covers a broad range of activities that contribute to the welfare of children. Such activities include the core activities of (i) care or activities that fulfill the survival needs of children, (ii) control or activities that appropriately discipline children, and (iii) development or activities that expand the potential of children (Hoghughi 2004). Clearly, the of parenting-practice is biased toward parents and children occupying the same space and sharing the same time. Indeed, society prescribes parenting standards that reinforce certain spatial and temporal conditions.

However, the parenting practices of transnational families do not follow the prescribed spatial and temporal conditions of parenting. As such, even with the consequent increase in the number of transnational families due to the volume of Filipinos seeking better opportunities abroad, and the advent of new technologies that enable migrant parents to engage in more involved mediated parenting, society is still wary of the reality of transnational families because it violates society's normative prescription of the "right" kind of family (Parreñas 2005a). Consequently, transnational families are not only struggling with the everyday reality of uncertainty and separation, but they are also perpetually struggling with their families' dissonance with society's normative prescription of what a family is and how a family should be (Pernia et al. 2014).

On a basic level, the spatial and temporal conditions of the supposed right kind of family underscore the daily routines of intimacy that characterise the collective experience of family members (Parreñas 2005a). Understandably, it is easier for family members to carry out the daily routines of family intimacy when they spend time together and share space. However, geographic separation of transnational family members limits their shared time and space, so much so that members generally spend more time physically apart than together (Parreñas 2005a).

On a deeper level, the spatial and temporal conditions reflect the gendered normative prescription of the right kind of family. According to Parreñas (2005a):

> In Philippine contemporary society…[t]he modern nuclear family with a breadwinning father and a nurturing mother is the right kind of family. Women nurture and men discipline. Fathers earn income for the family and mothers can choose to supplement it. Mothers manage and budget households, yet they always manage to defer major decisions of the family to fathers. (p. 34)

Thus, while society is generally wary of the reality of transnational families, it is more reticent when the mothers are the ones migrating abroad to earn for the family (Parreñas 2005a, 2008). Indeed, society is circumspect about migrant mothers because they defy society's gendered spatial and temporal expectations. When mothers leave, they not only become the breadwinners of the family, conventionally the role of fathers, but also become spatially and temporally constrained from carrying out their socially prescribed nurturing role. In contrast, fathers who leave their families for overseas employment do not bear the same yoke. Migrant mothers thus live with the sociopsychological burden of the spatial and temporal dissonance of their parenting in their daily lives (Pernia et al. 2014).

Conceptual Bases of the Paradoxes in Mediated Parenting Experiences

Mick and Fournier (1998) defined paradox as something that is "both X and not-X at the same time" (p. 125). Applied in the context of technology, the concept of technology paradox recognises that technological experience could be concurrently favorable and unfavorable wherein positive mediated experiences could coexist with negative ones. It also acknowledges that technological experiences may present binary opposites at the same time or shift between them from time to time (Jarvenpaa and Lang 2005; Mick and Fournier 1998).

Jarvenpaa and Lang (2005) described eight mobile technology paradoxes, and some of these paradoxes are analogous to the eight central paradoxes that Mick and Fournier (1998) previously identified (Table 9.1).

The paradoxes listed below reflect the good and the bad that could simultaneously ensue in mediated experiences. Such dialectic tension in mediated experiences could generate sociopsychological burdens among technology adopters. Thus, aside from investigating the paradox in mediated experiences, Mick and Fournier (1998) likewise explored the behavioral strategies that technology adopters observe to cope with dissonance. They discovered that technology adopters engage in pre-acquisition avoidance strategies (i.e., ignore, refuse, delay), pre-acquisition confrontational strategies (i.e., pretest, buying heuristics, extended decision making, extended warranty/maintenance construct), consumption avoidance strategies (i.e., neglect, abandonment, distancing), and consumption confrontational strategies (i.e., accommodation, partnering, mastering) (Mick and Fournier 1998, p. 133).

Table 9.1 Technology paradoxes

Central paradoxes of technological products Mick and Fournier (1998, p. 126)	Mobile technology paradoxes Jarvenpaa and Lang (2005, p. 10)
Freedom/enslavement	Independence/dependence
Competence/incompetence	Competence/incompetence
Control/chaos	Empowerment/enslavement
Fulfills/creates needs	Fulfills needs/creates needs
Engaging/disengaging	Engaging/disengaging
Efficiency/inefficiency	Planning/improvisation
New/obsolete	Public/private
Assimilation/isolation	Illusion/disillusion

As the dimensions of space and time are integral in examining and understanding the occurrence of technology paradoxes, the present study adopts these dimensions in exploring the paradoxes that Singapore-based Filipino migrant mothers experience in their mediated parenting. As new media and technologies abate the constraints of space and time, mediated experiences that take place anywhere in the "space of flows" (Castells 2010, p. 407) and anytime in "timeless time" (Castells 2010, p. 460) could exhibit paradoxes. With regard to the independence/dependence paradox, Jarvenpaa and Lang (2005) explained that communication technology use enables people to connect independent of space and time. However, this form of independence coincides with dependence on communication technology. In relation to the competence/incompetence paradox, Jarvenpaa and Lang (2005) argued that while communication technology use allows people to feel that they can competently perform their tasks unencumbered by space and time, the assistance of communication technology in the performance of tasks engenders a certain sense of incompetence as well. With respect to the empowerment/enslavement paradox, Jarvenpaa and Lang (2005) observed that while communication technology use empowers people to feel in command regardless of space and time, communication technology also enslaves them as it permits unfettered social connections at virtually any time of the day and almost anywhere in the world.

Previous studies have also delved into the technology paradoxes experienced by users. In Horst's (2006) study of Jamaican transnational families, she uncovered that while some families viewed the mobile phone as a blessing, as it enables daily family transnational connections, others are more ambivalent as it also brings financial and psychological burdens (i.e., monetary cost of maintaining mobile phone credit, emotional toll associated with the prospect of being monitored). With regard to mothers, Lim and Soon (2010) found that information and communication technologies (ICTs) empowered Chinese and Korean mothers to carry out their maternal responsibilities anytime and anywhere, but effectively enslaved them to the task of mothering.

Method

This chapter presents findings drawn from the author's interviews of 32 Singapore-based Filipino migrant mothers. 2013 official government statistics rank Singapore third among the countries of deployment of overseas Filipino workers (Philippine Overseas Welfare Administration (POEA) 2013). In addition, a considerable number of Singapore-based Filipino migrant workers are women (POEA 2010). Hence, Singapore is a prime host country for studying Filipino transnational migrant mothers.

The women who participated in this study were employed in Singapore and had left behind at least one teenage child in the Philippines. They were recruited through referrals and upon obtaining their informed consent, they were interviewed once, from October 2010 to March 2011, at a time and location convenient to them. All interviews were audio-recorded and transcribed. The average age of these mothers was 39 where the youngest was 32 years old and the oldest 49. They had worked in Singapore for an average of 4.3 years and were employed across a range of white-collar occupations, from professionals, associate professionals, managers, sales and service workers, and clerical support workers. Half of the participants were domestic workers. With the exception of the domestic workers who had typically obtained a high school degree, the rest of the women had obtained at least a college degree.

Mobile phone ownership was universal among these migrant mothers and their families back home. The same could not be said about smartphones and internet-connected personal computers as during the time of the interview, only the white-collar mothers had access to these. As such, they were able to use a wider range of technology for their transnational parenting. Meanwhile, the migrant mothers who were domestic workers depended on their basic mobile phones for their transnational parenting. Of this latter go, a number also disclosed that they had limited computer skills, so they could not use internet-connected computers for their transnational parenting even if such devices were accessible to them.

Paradoxes in Filipino Migrant Mothers' Mobile Parenting Experiences

Mobile parenting is a reconfiguration of onsite parenting to remote parenting through mobile communication. It highlights the communicative character of parenting as migrant mothers, their children, and their children's caregivers narrate activities, exchange experiences, extend care, share concerns, express emotions, and articulate affections through mediated communication. As mobile parenting primarily depends on communication, migrant mothers should be able to engage their children and their children's caregivers to talk to them to get updates about their families, which will then guide these mothers in parenting proactively and appropriately.

The findings showed that paradoxes inhere in migrant mothers' use of mobile communication technology for parenting. Specifically, the paradoxes that were uncovered were understood in terms of (1) the technological circumstances of the paradox, which revolve around the spatial and temporal freedoms that mobile communication technologies facilitate, and (2) the social circumstances of the paradox, which center on the spatial and temporal conditions of parenting at the family and societal levels. Of the eight aforementioned paradoxes (Jarvenpaa and Lang 2005; Mick and Fournier 1998), the independence/dependence, competence/incompetence, and empowerment/enslavement paradoxes were the most salient.

Independence/Dependence Paradox

The mothers shared that the availability of advanced communication technologies made the decision to work and remain overseas tolerable. As noted by a participant who had been working in Singapore for 2 years noted:

> I'm working abroad because my family needs the income that I'm earning from working overseas. At the outset, I dreaded leaving the country because I knew that I would terribly miss my family. I also knew that my family would terribly miss me. However, the assurance of regular contact through mobile communication made leaving the country easier to bear. It also makes staying abroad more bearable. (Sales and service worker, 32 years old, two daughters)

This was a recurring sentiment among the migrant mothers interviewed as the spatial and temporal separation that transnational labor migration entails is especially challenging for family-oriented Filipinos. At the heart of it, the strong affective ties that bind Filipino families are the same affective ties that make leaving the family behind to work overseas emotionally trying to endure.

Society's normative prescription of the right kind of family stresses that shared daily experiences of family life, which necessitate physical and temporal coexistence, strengthen affective ties (Parreñas 2005a). Based on society's normative standards then, transnational migrant mothers and their families are at a disadvantage since they do not have the luxury of shared space and time. Opportunely, mobile communication offers transnational migrant mothers the possibility of sustaining affective connections regardless of space and time. Wilding (2006) wrote, "The use of ICTs is important for some transnational families in constructing or imagining a 'connected relationship', and enabling them to overlook their physical separation by time and space – even if only temporarily" (p. 132). The promise of perpetual contact (Katz and Aakhus 2002) and simultaneity (Paragas 2008) free migrant parents from spatial and temporal constraints as the use of mobile communication technologies allows them to remain connected and to share "virtual intimacies" (Wilding 2006, p. 125) with their families anytime and anywhere. One mother related:

> Although my daughter felt sad when she learned that I would be going away, she understood that our family needed the income that I would get from working abroad. Before I left, my daughter and I kept on reassuring each other that staying in touch is easy because we have mobile phones. (Domestic worker, 37 years old, one daughter and two sons)

As Uy-Tioco (2007) wrote, "technology makes physical presence less of a necessity" (p. 261). Parreñas (2001) refers to the use of communication media and technologies for maintaining and sustaining relationships among transnational family members as the "technological management of distance" (pp. 130–131).

In the case of sustaining emotional connections, mobile communication rendered affective ties to be independent of space and time. Accordingly, transnational migrant mothers are unchained from spatial-and-temporal-bound emotional ties. In effect, mobile communication offers migrant mothers more independence to stay abroad longer and thus generate more savings for the family (Paragas 2005). However, while migrant mothers' use of mobile communication technologies unfetters them to pursue affective ties transnationally, they consequently become dependent on the very same technology that frees them. This is the independence/dependence paradox in transnational migrant mothers' mobile parenting experience. Consistent with extant literature on transnational family communication (i.e., Aguilar et al. 2009; Cabanes and Acedera 2012; Madianou and Miller 2011, 2012b; Paragas 2005, 2008; Parreñas 2005a, b; San Pascual 2014a, b; Uy-Tioco 2007; Thomas and Lim 2011), the interviews revealed that Singapore-based Filipino migrant mothers are highly dependent on their mobile phone for sustaining strong emotional bonds with their families back home:

> I couldn't image what our family life would be without our mobile phones. (Domestic worker, 41 years old, one daughter)

Factors such as preference for newer forms of technology, accessibility of the technology, and skills in using the technology determine the migrant mothers' dependence on mobile phones. These factors echo the technological preconditions of access, affordability, and literacy that Madianou and Miller (2012a) identified. These mothers disclosed that the mobile phone is the most basic communication medium that they and their families must own to be able to manage their transnational separation. They elucidated that ownership and exclusive use of the device offer them privacy in communication and similarly enable them to monitor their overseas communication expenses.

While mobile phone ownership was universal among the migrant mothers interviewed, there were disparities in the habitual use of mobile communication technologies between the white-collar mothers and the domestic worker mothers. Since the former have access to a wider array of mobile-based and internet-based technologies, they are not overly dependent on mobile communication for their long-distance connection with their families. These mothers have replaced habitual sending of daily SMS with daily internet voice/video call. In contrast, the migrant mothers who are employed in domestic work only have access to basic mobile-based technologies; hence, these mothers could only depend on their mobile phone for their overseas connection with their families. They habitually send daily SMS to their children and engage in weekly mobile voice calls. Furthermore, they were also dependent on their mobile phone for their long-distance communication with their families because they divulged that they were not computer literate. Consequently, these mothers' dependence on mobile communication technologies came at a cost, especially for those earning lower incomes. They had to prudently manage their earnings to cover their living expenses, remittances, and regular long-distance communication expenses.

Nevertheless, the migrant mothers have accepted their consequent dependence on mobile communication in order to sustain their affective family ties. While mobile communication is not cost-free, they recognise that the price is reasonable considering the benefits they derive from its use. As such, in order to manage their dependence on mobile communication, these mothers engage in strategies that would fit their mobile communication needs and budget. In the case of the white-collar mothers, their access to a wider range of communication media and technologies allows them to engage in "polymedia" (Madianou and Miller 2012a, b) strategies as they can access a wider array of choices on which medium and technology to use to sustain their family connections. While the domestic worker mothers do not have the same breadth of access, they nonetheless engage in what the current author refers to as "polytechnology" strategies as these mothers choose from the technologies offered by their basic mobile phone to sustain their affective family ties.

Competence/Incompetence Paradox in Mobile Parenting

Society's normative prescription of the right kind of family emphasizes the spatial and temporal dimensions of shared daily family life experiences. By extension, society's normative prescription of the right kind of parenting stresses the spatial and temporal dimensions of parenting. However, mobile communication offers transnational migrant parents an opportunity to parent their children regardless of space and time. Thus, the use of mobile communication technologies for transnational parenting permits these migrant mothers to feel that they are still competently involved in the lives of their children.

Mobile parenting allows migrant mothers to maintain what Pertierra (2005), as quoted by Uy-Tioco (2007), referred to as "absent presence" (p. 259) wherein migrant mothers are able to perform long-distance caretaking and caregiving of their children. As one mother articulated:

> Even if I'm living apart from my children, it's like I'm still there. (Domestic worker, 37 years old, two sons)

This echoes the sentiment of one of the mother informants in Hondagneu-Sotelo and Avila's (1997) study when the mother expressed, "I'm here, but I'm there" (p. 558).

The interviews show that mobile parenting is not only motivated by the desire to sustain affective family ties but is also driven by the desire to secure the well-being of their children. Through mobile parenting, migrant mothers are able to extend their care, concern, love, and affection for their children despite the distance. In their habitual mobile communication, Singapore-based Filipino migrant mothers extend their care and concern for their children by discussing matters related to their children's welfare. For instance, mothers frequently ask their children how they are and how their day has been. A migrant mother, whose daughter studies and lives in the city, narrated:

> My daughter lives away from the family because she studies in the city. So apart from my regular overseas contact with my husband and my younger daughter, I also frequently contact my older daughter so I could personally know how she is doing. (Domestic worker, 39 years old, two daughters)

This way, the migrant mothers explained that if their children are not okay, they could still guide them on what to do even if they could not be physically present to care for them in person. Another migrant mother shared:

> When my daughter got sick, I advised her to take herbal remedy and I called every 30 minutes to ask how she was feeling. (Domestic worker, 37 years old, one daughter and two sons)

All the migrant mothers interviewed also mentioned that they discuss matters about school in their attempt at mobile parenting. They also remarked that they try to actively help their children with their homework and school projects. Moreover, migrant mothers with children who are about to enter tertiary level education discuss school and course prospects with their children. For instance, one mother recounted:

> When my daughter was about to enter college, we often talked about the courses that she could possibly take. I gave her advice but I let her decide. (CAD drafter, 44 years old, two daughters and one son)

Additionally, as the interviews were conducted among migrant mothers with teenage children, these mothers also encourage their adolescent children to talk to them about their initiation to romance. In fact, while some mothers are open to their teenage children engaging in romantic relationship, others downright discouraged it. Nonetheless, these mothers are careful not to strongly impose their position so that their children would see them as open-minded and would feel comfortable in sharing their romantic life with them. A number of mothers even disclosed that they strive for friendship with their teenage children. This way, their children would feel comfortable in sharing their initiation into romance:

> I am friends with my daughter so she is comfortable in talking to me about the guys courting her. Since I get information directly from her, I have the opportunity to guide her on her initiation to romance. (Sales Consultant, 36 years old, one daughter)

> My son and I are buddies. I open up about my dating life with him so he would also do the same, so he would also feel comfortable in sharing his dating life with me. (Freelance make-up artist and lounge singer, 34 years old, two sons)

Moreover, in their habitual mobile communication, these mothers also convey their love and affection for their children. Thus, it is also usual for these women to constantly exchange statements of "I love you" and "I miss you" in their conversations with their children. As both parties could not perform physical expressions of love and affection during migration, these vocal articulations are even more important. According to Aguilar et al. (2009), "Even simple greetings… signified a relationship that remained valued despite the distance" (p. 207). A mother shared:

> Before we end our phone call, we keep on saying "I love you", "I miss you" repeatedly without us knowing that we have already spent two to three minutes just doing so. (Administrative Executive, 32 years old, one daughter)

There are also migrant mothers who disclosed that they are more expressive of their feelings now that they are living apart:

We're sweeter with each other now. Perhaps the distance drew us closer together, ironic isn't it? We're now more expressive of our feelings than before. (Operations Executive, 35 years old, one son and one daughter)

Yet, at the back of these mothers' minds, they still hold the notion that nothing less than physically present parenting could bring about competent parenting (Parreñas 2001, 2005a, b; Sobritchea 2007). As society prescribes mothers to personally administer childcare, it is common for migrant mothers to feel that they are not doing a good job as mothers because they are not physically around their children to personally care for them. Thus, the spatial and temporal conditions of society's normative prescription on the right kind of parenting generate feelings of incompetence among migrant mothers that the kind of parenting that they can afford to extend given their transnational situation is far from ideal. This is the competence/incompetence paradox in transnational migrant mothers' mobile parenting experience. While mobile communication allows these migrant mothers to feel that they are still competently involved in the lives of their children regardless of space and time, the deeply rooted spatial and temporal standards of the right kind of parenting hold them back from considering their brand of parenting as adequate. Thus, the dissonance engenders sociopsychological burden among migrant mothers. As one lamented:

Sometimes I feel like I'm a failure as a mother because I'm not with them. But what choice do I have? (Office/Production Administrator, 34 years old, one daughter and one son)

Almost all the migrant mothers interviewed expressed that they are working overseas primarily to finance their children's education. A mother explained:

My husband and I want our kids to experience a life better than the life we experienced and education is key to that. We couldn't depend on the income that we get back home so I have to work here to support our kids' education. (Domestic worker, 39 years old, two daughters)

While working overseas to finance their children's education is an honorable act of parenting, the migrant mothers feel that financially providing for the family is not enough. One emphatically expressed:

That's the curse of a mother working abroad, you are a mother financially but you are not a mother physically. (Domestic worker, 37 years old, two sons)

These migrant mothers could not help but feel that it is a toss-up between fulfilling the nurturing function of financially providing for their children's needs and that of personally administering care for their children. Thus, nuggets of doubt exist among the mothers on whether their decision to leave their families to be able to better provide for them justifies their absence from day-to-day family life. Furthermore, there are also feelings of uncertainty as to whether their remote parenting truly enables them to be a parent to their children and whether mediated parenting effectively substitutes for onsite parenting. Besides, there are also left-behind children who are wary of their transnational family separation and the benefit of transnational communication in managing the distance (Madianou and

Miller 2011). As Madianou and Miller (2011) observed, "children are significantly more ambivalent about the consequences of transnational communication" (p. 457).

Mobile parenting breaks spatial and temporal barriers through mobile communication. Given that mobile parenting is hinged on the ability to communicate, the migrant mothers also experience the competence/incompetence paradox whenever they find the act of interpersonal communication with their children and their children's caregivers difficult. Some migrant mothers disclosed that they feel incompetent when they could not properly express themselves. Some of them also shared that they feel inadequate when they could not find the right words to say. As Sobritchea (2007) explained, "The effort to communicate their love for their children was often hamstrung by their own inability to "find the right words" and "the right time to do it"" (p. 186).

Some of them also related that they feel incompetent in communicating with their children whenever they have to deal with conflicts and tension. A mother shared:

> It is such a joy to talk to my kids during happy moments but it is such a task to talk to them when we have disagreements. (Domestic worker, 37 years old, one daughter and two sons)

Another migrant mother described the emotional volatility and rebellious tendencies of her 16-year-old daughter. She related the difficulties she experienced in dealing with her daughter because she is unsure of how her daughter would react to more aggressive forms of admonishment.

These mothers also experience the competence/incompetence paradox whenever they encounter the limitations of mediated communication:

> When my daughter got sick, I could not really do anything aside from talk. I felt so helpless. If I were there, then I could personally take care of my daughter. But I couldn't afford to go home. I felt so inadequate as a mother. (Domestic worker, 37 years old, one daughter and two sons)

Thus, mothers who could manage to return home during emergencies would do so:

> When my son got his girlfriend pregnant, he didn't know how he would tell his father and he was also afraid of how his father would react to the news. I had to take an emergency leave so I could be there to mediate between my son and my husband. (Domestic worker, 37 years old, one son and one daughter)

While these mothers are aware of the scope of parenting that mediated communication affords them, they recognise that it is the situational limitation imposed by their migration-led separation, not the technological limitation inherent in mobile communication, which truly hinders them from fully parenting their children. Hence, while these mothers are aware that transnational communication is not without deficiencies, they categorically expressed their satisfaction and even amazement at how mediated communication facilitates their reaching out to their children.

Parreñas (2005b) observed that, "The children who receive constant communication from migrant parents are less likely to feel a gap in intergenerational relations" (p. 105). She (2005a, b) found that care by mothers across distance eases the burden of migration among left-behind children and that children can better cope with the changes if they have assurances of their mother's love. Still, she (2005a) counseled that nurturing and caring should not be exclusively expected from mothers and advised that institutions of social learning should be careful not to propagate gendered family roles that confine the role of breadwinning to fathers and the caregiving duty to mothers. This way, children will be exposed to a more dynamic view of family and family roles, and this will thus make adjustments to transnational family life less difficult.

Empowerment/Enslavement Paradox in Mobile Parenting

Parenting covers a broad range of nurture, control, and development activities intended to ensure the well-being of children (Hoghughi 2004). The Singapore-based Filipino migrant mothers interviewed acknowledged that parenting is best carried out onsite because parenting is intrinsically a visual and tactile activity:

> As a parent, I would like to personally monitor what is happening to my children and I would like to personally take care of them. (Course Superintendent, 42 years old, two sons and two daughters)

While migrant mothers cannot perform onsite parenting, mobile communication technologies empower them to maintain what Katz and Aakhus (2002) described as being "physically mobile, but socially "in touch"" (p. 301). Madianou and Miller (2011) observed that migrant mothers view their ability to micromanage the care of their children through mobile communication as empowering. Uy-Tioco (2007) wrote that, "Cell phone technology has empowered these women, creating new ways to 'mother' their children across time and space" (p. 253). As one mother articulated:

> It's hard, but through communication, I can still be a mother to my children. (Domestic worker, 43 years old, two sons)

The migrant mothers strive to perform remote nurturing functions through mobile parenting when they prompt their children with questions such as "Kamusta ka?" ("How are you?") and "Kamusta ang araw mo?" ("How was your day?") in their attempts to monitor their children's welfare and safety. They also get updates about their children from their children's caregivers. In this manner, the mothers feel that they could still be involved in their children's nurturing despite the distance. Additionally, these mothers are also fond of asking questions such as "Kumain ka na ba?" ("Have you eaten?") or "Ano kinain mo?" ("What have you eaten?") to express that they are still concerned about the seemingly mundane events in their children's daily lives.

The migrant mothers also endeavor to carry out offsite control functions through mobile parenting when they remind their children of their boundaries. For instance, they remind their teenage children about the rules that they have to observe with regard to romance. Furthermore, since sex is a touchy matter for discussion in the predominantly conservative Roman Catholic culture of the Philippines, Filipino parents do not typically discuss matters concerning premarital sex with their children. As such, when the migrant mothers talk about the restrictions that their children should observe when it comes to romance, they usually do so in the context of reminding their teens of the consequence of early pregnancy and its subsequent effect on the completion of their studies and on their future:

> I remind my daughter that she succeeded in starting high school early and if she keeps it up, she'll be able to graduate early as well. I tell her that having a boyfriend could only distract her from finishing ahead. I tell her that after she graduates, then she could do anything that she wants. (Administrative Executive, 32 years old, one daughter)

At the same time however, there are mothers who are more upfront in talking about sex:

> I wanted to remind my daughter about her boundaries when it comes to engaging in romantic relationship. I didn't know how to open the discussion on avoiding premarital sex because it is not a topic that Filipino parents usually talk about with their children. Then, I got an idea on how to talk to my daughter about it after I heard my Western employers giving their daughters reminders about sex. So one time, I called up my daughter specifically to talk about avoiding premarital sex. (Domestic worker, 33 years old, one daughter and one son)

In addition, the mothers also strive to carry out remote control functions through mobile parenting when they impose discipline. However, they admitted that they are more careful in administering reproof as such could lead to misunderstandings:

> I exercise caution when I discipline my child. I make sure that my child understands where I'm coming from to avoid any untoward misunderstandings. (Administrative Executive, 32 years old, one daughter)

> We are already living apart so I don't want to create any emotional distance between us. (Sales Consultant, 36 years old, one daughter)

These quotes reflect Aguilar et al's. (2009) findings that migrant parents tend to be "hesitant disciplinarians" (p. 262).

Apart from remote nurturing and control functions, the migrant mothers also attempt to perform development functions through mobile parenting when they try to be actively involved in their children's education:

> I keep telling my eldest son to study hard so he could succeed in life. (Domestic worker, 43 years old, two sons)

There are also migrant mothers who relayed how they would tutor their kids while on mobile voice call:

> I plug my earphones and use my mobile phone's hands-free capability when I have to talk to my family while working. My employers are not bothered as long as my overseas calls do not get in the way of accomplishing my daily chores. There are times when I'm preparing dinner and, at the same time, I'm tutoring my kids. (Domestic worker, 39 years old, two daughters)

Migrant mothers also celebrate the successes of their kids in school through mobile parenting. A mother narrated her experience of calling her family during the graduation ceremony of one of her children:

> I couldn't go home at that time but my family promised me that they would call me up so I could join them when they come up on stage. So my husband called me just before our son's name was called. Though I could only faintly hear what was going on, I felt that I was also with my family while my son received his diploma and award. (Domestic worker, 43 years old, two sons)

Some mothers also related that they have the mobile number of their children's teachers so that they could get in touch with them whenever needs arise:

> Once, I got an emergency call from my daughter and she told me that her school received a bomb threat. I told her to follow her teacher's instructions and not to worry about the things she left in the classroom. Then I called her school's guidance counselor to ask what was going on and to get assurance that the school is keeping all the kids safe. (Assistant Teacher, 42 years old, two sons and one daughter)

However, while mobile parenting empowers transnational migrant mothers to perform offsite nurturing, control, and development functions, it also enslaves them to society' gendered parenting standards. Devasahayam and Yeoh (2007) wrote, "The reproductive burden and the care of children in the domestic sphere remain firmly women's work – not men's – even in situations when mothering practices have to be fashioned in transnational terms at a great distance" (p. 21).

In effect, while mobile parenting freed migrant mothers from space-and-time constraints to perform remote parenting, it likewise freed the enactment of gendered parenting norms from space-and-time constraints. Although mobile parenting empowers migrant mothers to parent their children beyond financial provision, it also shackles them as it enacts the multiple gendered burdens of mothers. Hence, mobile parenting "reinforces traditional roles in a patriarchal system" (Uy-Tioco 2007, p. 264).

Nevertheless, while it may appear that mediated parenting perpetuates gendered parenting norms, for the migrant mothers interviewed, they simply want to parent their children. Cheng (2004) wrote,

> For the millions of migrant women..., the issue of motherhood is not about male dominance, the public-private dichotomy, unequal gender division of labor, double shift, or struggle for individual autonomy. For them, they cannot mother their children the conventional way because economic deterioration and family survival compel them to seek overseas employment... In short, their fundamental concern is the deprivation of their right to motherhood (p. 136).

In order to ease the emotional burden of labor migration-led separation, there is a need for society to reconfigure its construction of parenting. Expanding the definition of parenting to welcome transnational parenting would be more inclusive of families who are physically but not affectively apart. Moreover, it is also imperative for society to reassess its primarily gendered construction of parental role expectations so that families can better cope with the challenges and limitations imposed by transnational labor migration (Parreñas 2005a).

Conclusion

Communication is a vital part of mobile parenting. While mobile parenting does not entirely compensate for the loss of physical presence, it is a viable means of channeling an offsite presence. Through mobile parenting, the Singapore-based Filipino migrant mothers are able to reach out to their children, maintain their relationship with them, and practice parenting responsibilities regardless of space and time.

The dimensions of space and time are integral in examining the independence/dependence, competence/incompetence, and empowerment/enslavement paradoxes that the Singapore-based Filipino migrant mothers experience when they engage in mobile parenting. These paradoxes were understood in terms of the spatial and temporal freedom that mobile communication technologies facilitate as well as the spatial and temporal conditions of parenting. The interviews with these migrant mothers revealed that when they engage in mobile parenting, they experience independence, competence, and empowerment and, at the same time, they experience dependence, incompetence, and enslavement. In other words, the mobile parenting experiences of migrant mothers are not entirely celebratory as positive mediated experiences coexist with negative ones.

This study, however, has several limitations, which future transnational migration and family communication research may address. First, this study directed its attention to the mediated experiences of Filipino migrant mothers. While mothers constitute a significant segment of Filipinos in diaspora, it would also be interesting to find out the paradoxes in the mediated parenting experiences of migrant fathers. As society prescribes a distinct set of gendered roles for Filipino fathers (Medina 2001; Parreñas 2008), their experienced paradoxes may be different from those that migrant mothers experience. Aside from migrant parents, an examination of the mediated experiences of children and caregivers would further expand our understanding of technology paradox from the context of left-behind family members. Second, this study focused on migrant mothers who are based in Singapore, and the paradoxes in their mobile parenting experiences may be different from migrant parents who are land-based or sea-based, e.g., seamen. For instance, Singapore is on the same time zone as the Philippines and the parallel day-and-night cycle of migrant parents and left-behind children may consequently heighten the temporal dimension of their perpetual contact. Moreover, the communication environment of Singapore-based migrant parents may be different from that of migrant parents who are based in other countries. Based on the interviews, Singapore offers a relatively flexible environment for migrant parents to engage in long-distance communication with their families back home. Finally, this study analyzed interviews that were conducted at a time where access and use of smartphones were only concentrated among white-collar mothers. Thus, it would be interesting to discover how the expansion of access to smartphones among migrant parents and their left-behind children, if and when it occurs, transforms the dynamics in their mediated experiences.

We live in an imperfect world where the good coexists with the bad. In the case of technology paradoxes, human-technology interaction reveals whether the value of experiencing a particular technology favors one end of the spectrum over the other. For the Singapore-based Filipino migrant mothers, while mobile parenting engenders paradoxes in mediated experiences, it is nonetheless the best response to the situation imposed by transnational labor migration. Therefore, for these migrant mothers, even if negative experiences coexist with positive one, these mothers can still reach out to their children, maintain their relationship with them, and practice their parenting responsibilities regardless of space and time.

References

Aguilar Jr, F. V., Peñalosa, J. E. Z., Liwanag, T. B. T., Cruz, R. S., & Melendrez, J. M. (2009). *Maalwang buhay: Family, overseas migration, and cultures of relatedness in Barangay Paraiso*. Quezon City: Ateneo de Manila Univaguilarersity Press.

Asis, M. M. B., Huang, S., & Yeoh, B. S. A. (2004). When the light of the home is abroad: Unskilled female migration and the Filipino family. *Singapore Journal of Tropical Geography, 25*(2), 198–215. doi: 10.1111/j.0129-7619.2004.00182.x.

Cabanes, J. V. A., & Acedera, K. A. F. (2012). Of mobile phones and mother-fathers: Calls, text messages, and conjugal power relations in mother-away Filipino families. *New Media & Society, 14*(6), 916–930. doi: 10.1177/1461444811435397.

Castells, M. (2010). *The rise of the network society* (2nd ed.). West Sussex: Wiley and Blackwell.

Cheng, S. A. (2004). Right to mothering: Motherhood as a transborder concern in the age of globalization. *Journal of Association for Research on Mothering, 6*(1), 135–144. Retrieved from http://pi.library.yorku.ca.libproxy1.nus.edu.sg/ojs/index.php/jarm/article/viewFile/4891/4085

Chu, W., & Yang, S. (2006). Mobile phones and new migrant workers in South China village: An initial analysis of the interplay between the "social" and the "technological". In P. Law, L. Fortunati, & S. Yang (Eds.), *New technologies in global societies* (pp. 221–244). Singapore: World Scientific Publishing Co. Pvt. Ltd.

Devasahayam, T. W., & Yeoh, B. S. A (2007). Asian women negotiating work challenges and family commitments. In T. W. Devasahayam & B. S. A. Yeoh (Eds.), *Working and mothering in Asia: Images, ideologies and identities* (pp. 3–26). Singapore: NUS Press.

Hoghughi, M. (2004). Handbook of parenting: An introduction. In M. Hoghughi & N. Long (Eds.), *Theory and research for practice* (pp. 1–18). London: Sage Publications.

Hondagneu-Sotelo, P., & Avila, E. (1997). I'm here, but I'm there: The meanings of Latina transnational motherhood. *Gender & Society, 11*(5), 548–571. doi: 10.1177/089124397011005003.

Horst, H. A. (2006). The blessing and burdens of communication: Cellphones in Jamaican transnational social fields. *Global Networks, 6*(2), 143–159.

Jarvenpaa, S. L., & Lang, K. R. (2005). Managing the paradoxes of mobile technology. *Information Systems Management, 22*(4), 7–23.

Katz, J. E., & Aakhus, M. (Eds.) (2002). *Perpetual contact: Mobile communication, private talks, public performance*. Cambridge: Cambridge University Press.

Lim, S. S., & Soon, C. (2010). The influence of social and cultural factors on mothers' domestication of household ICTs – Experiences of Chinese and Korean women. *Telematics and Informatics, 27*(3), 205–216.

Madianou, M., & Miller, D. (2011). Mobile phone parenting: Reconfiguring relationships between Filipina migrant mothers and their left-behind children. *New Media and Society, 13*(3), 457–470. doi: 10.1177/1461444810393903.

Madianou, M., & Miller, D. (2012a). Polymedia: Toward a new theory of digital media in interpersonal communication. *International Journal of Cultural Studies, 16*(2), 169–187. doi: 10.1177/1367877912452486.
Madianou, M., & Miller, D. (2012b). *Migration and new media: Transnational families and polymedia*. Oxon/New York: Routledge.
Medina, B. T. G. (2001). *The Filipino family* (2nd ed.). Quezon City: The University of the Philippines Press.
Mick, D. G., & Fournier, S. (1998). Paradoxes of technology: Consumer cognizance, emotions, and coping strategies. *The Journal of Consumer Research, 25*(2), 123–143.
Paragas, F. (2005). Migrant mobiles: Cellular telephony, transnational spaces, and the Filipino diaspora. In K. Nyiri (Ed.), *A sense of place: The global and the local in mobile communication* (pp. 241–249). Vienna: Die Deutsche Bibliothek.
Paragas, F. (2008). Migrant workers and mobile phones: Technological, temporal, and spatial simultaneity. In R. Ling & S. W. Campbell (Eds.), *The reconstruction of space and time: Mobile communications practices* (pp. 39–65). New Brunswick: Transaction Publishers.
Parreñas, R. S. (2001). *Servants of globalization: Women, migration, and domestic work*. Stanford: Stanford University Press.
Parreñas, R. S. (2005a). *Children of global migration: Transnational families and gendered woes*. Stanford: Stanford University Press.
Parreñas, R. S. (2005b). Long distance intimacy: Class, gender and intergenerational relations between mothers and children in Filipino transnational families. *Global Networks, 5*(4), 317–336. doi: 10.1111/j.1471-0374.2005.00122.x.
Parreñas, R. S. (2008). Transnational fathering: Gendered conflicts, distant disciplining and emotional gaps. *Journal of Ethnic and Migration Studies, 34*(7), 1057–1072. doi: 10.1080/13691830802230356.
Pernia, E. M., Pernia, E. E., Ubias, J. L., & San Pascual, M. R. S. (2014). *International migration, remittances, and economic development in the Philippines*. Manila: De La Salle University Publishing House.
Pertierra, R. (2005). Mobile phones, identity and discursive intimacy. *Human Technology: An Interdisciplinary Journal on Humans in ICT Environments, 1*(1), 23–44.
Philippine Overseas Employment Administration. (2010). *OFW deployment per country per skill*. Mandaluyong City: Philippine Overseas Employment Administration.
Philippine Overseas Employment Administration. (2013). *Compendium of OFW statistics 2009–2013*. Mandaluyong City: Philippine Overseas Employment Administration.
San Pascual, M. R. S. (2014a). Living through the parameters of technology: Filipino mothers in Diaspora and their mediated parenting experiences. *Plaridel Journal, 11*(1), 35–62.
San Pascual, M. R. S. (2014b). Mobile parenting and global mobility: The case of Filipino migrant mothers. In X. Xu (Ed.), *Interdisciplinary mobile media and communications: Social, political and economic implications* (pp. 194–212). Pennsylvania: IGI Global.
Sobritchea, C. I. (2007). Constructions of mothering: The experience of female Filipino overseas workers. In T. W. Devasahayam & B. S. A. Yeoh (Eds.), *Working and mothering in Asia: Images, ideologies and identities* (pp. 173–194). Singapore: NUS Press.
Thomas, M., & Lim, S. S. (2011). On maids and mobile phones: ICT use by female migrant workers in Singapore and its policy implications. In J. E. Katz (Ed.), *Mobile communication: Dimensions of social policy* (pp. 175–190). New Brunswick: Transaction Publishers.
Uy-Tioco, C. (2007). Overseas Filipino workers and text messaging: Reinventing transnational mothering. *Continuum: Journal of Media & Cultural Studies, 21*(2), 253–265. doi: 10.1080/10304310701269081.
Vertovec, S. (2004). Cheap calls: The social glue of migrant transnationalism. *Global Networks, 4*(2), 219–224. doi: 10.1111/j.1471-0374.2004.00088.x.
Wilding, R. (2006). 'Virtual' intimacies? Families communicating across transnational contexts. *Global Networks, 6*(2), 125–142. doi: 10.1111/j.1471-0374.2006.00137.x.

Chapter 10
The Value of the Life Course Perspective in the Design of Mobile Technologies for Older Adults

Pin Sym Foong

Abstract In gerontology and geriatrics, the life course perspective is a well-established and fruitful approach to the study of older adults. In this chapter, a case is made for the inclusion of the life course perspective in the field of human-computer interaction (HCI) for older adults. A quadrant analysis on the axes of age and wellness was conducted. This resulted in the creation of a Gerotech clock depicting four phases of older adults as users of mobile computers – maintaining, compensating, coping and caring. Each of these phases was examined for ways in which the life course perspective could inform the study of older adults.

Three potential research areas were uncovered. Firstly, the transition from older adults being relatively mobile to having impairments was identified as a rich space for the identification of choice points in which older adults adapt their use of mobile technologies. Secondly, caregivers of older adults were identified as a poorly understood user group that offered a critical challenge to the long-standing HCI concepts of *user* and *primary user*. Thirdly, with the use of demographic and epidemiological data in Singapore, the complex of challenges that family caregivers of older adults face was explained. Informed by the life course perspective, a research agenda that seeks to understand the technological needs of older adults and their caregivers within the site of the family is proposed.

Keywords Gerotech clock • HCI • Gerontology • Older adults • Caregivers • Mobile technologies • Impairments

> The ageing population is unprecedented, pervasive and enduring.
> United Nations (UN) report on *World Population Ageing, 1950–2050* (2002)

While much has been said about the ageing population in many developed countries, the statement above brings one more element into the mix – the notion that an ageing population is the new normal and that, barring catastrophic events, 'the aged

---

P.S. Foong (✉)
National University of Singapore, Singapore
e-mail: pinsym@u.nus.edu

© Springer Science+Business Media Dordrecht 2016
S.S. Lim (ed.), *Mobile Communication and the Family*, Mobile Communication in Asia: Local Insights, Global Implications,
DOI 10.1007/978-94-017-7441-3_10

we will always have with us' (Paraphrased from the Bible, Matthew 26:11, New International Version).

The discipline of human-computer interaction (HCI) has made significant contributions to the development of technologies that can offer geriatric care and support. However, in light of current realities, HCI needs to go beyond seeing older adults merely as a user group with challenging characteristics. Instead, there is a need to broaden HCI's narrow conceptualisation of the elderly by going beyond the discipline to survey existing ageing – related research – and to draw on established methodology. In this regard, the life course perspective, a commonly used approach to study the ageing process in geriatrics and gerontology, may offer a critical frame of reference for HCI.

Stoller and Gibson define the life course perspective as one that 'highlights the ways in which people's location in the social system, the historical period in which they live, and their unique personal biographies shape the experience of old age' (2000, p. 19). The purpose of this chapter is to introduce and consider the potential value of the life course perspective as a method to develop a richer understanding of an increasingly salient aspect of ageing in urbanised, developed countries – the use and relevance of mobile technology. Through an explanation and application of the life course perspective in Singapore's context, this chapter aims to establish the relevant themes at the intersection of the life course perspective and HCI, particularly in the area of mobile technologies. It also identifies gaps in the research for older adults and mobile technologies with a proposal for future research directions that have both social and academic significance.

The data used in this chapter is from studies on the Singapore population, unless otherwise stated.

Connecting HCI and the Life Course Perspective

The study of HCI has its roots in human factors engineering from the 1970s. Using the behavioural and empirical tenets of cognitive psychology, it measured the human response to various devices and endeavoured to change the interface to improve efficiency and efficacy (Benyon et al. 2005).

Since then, the problem in HCI, particularly in mobile HCI, has widened to encompass the experience of technology, predictive factors for adoption and, more broadly, the exploration of technology as 'practice' (Pacey 1983). The widespread adoption of mobile technology has fuelled this mode of problematisation. As described by ex-Nokia developer Barbara Ballard (2007), mobile technologies have the following features – mobility, connectivity and the 'carry principle', referring to technologies that are small and ever present. Smartphones and tablet-sized computing devices, with their mobility-friendly form factors, contribute to the ubiquity of mobile technology. Coupled with sensor-enabled devices or haptic extensions, these portable computers can become pervasive – a part of everyday life and used for the most mundane of tasks. Finally, when linked to home, city- and countrywide network infrastructure, mobile phones can be ambient technologies, collecting data that in turn is used to shape our experience of the world around us. As a response to the development of mobile technologies, researchers have readily accepted a shift in methodology – ethnography and ethnographic analysis, with their pragmatic focus on experience and felt-life, are now accepted methods in the design of user-centred computing systems.

Ageing nations with their growing numbers of elderly, accompanied by the rising penetration of mobile technology across all demographic groups, have presented new challenges to mobile technology researchers. These challenges tend to centre on healthcare issues, from supporting age-related impairments to dealing with disabilities and even death and dying. Hitherto, the response to such challenges has primarily been through these lenses: cognitive, context aware, situational, ecological and systemic – each reflecting different schools of thought in HCI research. What these diverse lenses have in common is a focus on ageing adults as a group, treated as distinct from other age groups in their abilities and motivations for the use of mobile technology. In the remainder of this chapter, I will argue that this perspective is limiting, in that it does not acknowledge the nature of ageing as an active, ongoing process. Researchers who adopt the group perspective often find it challenging to account for the wild heterogeneity within the user group caused by age-linked pathologies and by older users' 'unique personal biographies'. Whenever older adults are treated as a homogenous group, researchers may overlook some of the nuanced perspectives and insights that a lifespan-oriented approach can offer. I propose that with the, as the UN (2002) puts it, 'unprecedented, pervasive and enduring' nature of ageing, the time seems right to draw certain epistemic threads together, so as to forge a fruitful approach that productively incorporates the life course perspective into the field of HCI for older adults.

The Life Course Perspective

Hutchison (2010, p. 30) identifies the major concerns of the life course perspective as a gerontological approach that studies the following six subjects:

1. The interplay of human lives and historical time: Individual and family development must be understood in historical context.
2. The timing of lives: Particular roles and behaviours are associated with particular age groups, based on biological, psychological, social and spiritual age.
3. The existence of linked or interdependent lives: Human lives are interdependent, and the family is the primary arena for experiencing and interpreting wider historical, cultural and social phenomena.
4. Human agency in making choices: The individual life course is constructed by the choices and actions individuals take within the opportunities and constraints of history and social circumstances.
5. The diversity in life course trajectories: There is much diversity in life course pathways, due to cohort variations, social class, culture, gender and individual agency.

6. Developmental risk and protection: Experiences with one life transition have an impact on subsequent transitions and events and may either protect the life course trajectory or put it at risk.

While it is neither a theory nor a framework, the life course perspective is an illuminating approach that exhorts researchers to take into account the entire lifespan when studying ageing phenomena, rather than to just focus on the current state of affairs.

When applied to medicine, the life course perspective steers researchers towards understanding how past health behaviours and conditions can change an older adult's current responses to a health challenge. From these findings, public health measures are constructed to target key choices or trajectories of risk. The case of respiratory disease by Ben-Shlomo and Kuh (2002, p. 286) is a good illustration of the application of the life course approach in medicine. For newborns, poor growth in utero and weak lung development can put the infant on a life trajectory for respiratory infections. Repeated infections over time become a factor for rapid lung decline in adult lung disease. The effect of childhood experiences can be exacerbated by poor adult socio-economic status, living in an area with poor air quality or working in hazardous jobs. Hence, when making public health policies, targeting choice behaviours is indicated – for example, the good management of childhood chest illness is possibly preventive, as is managing air quality for adults at risk of lung disease.

How does a lifespan approach in medicine transfer to research in HCI?

Currently, items 1, 2 and 3 on the list above already exist to differing extents in HCI research. For example, item 1 resonates with studies that look at cohort effects on older adults' adoption of technology. For example, Wilkowska and Ziefle (2009) found that previous training at work and technical self-confidence greatly influenced acceptance of technology among the older adults. In general, however, HCI research does not account for collective historical events, only personal. Item 2, the timing of lives, refers to the identification of certain roles and behaviours with certain age groups. With regard to ageing adults and HCI, the link between ageing, technology and grandparenting has been the subject of some studies (e.g. Vutborg et al. 2010), as has been ageing, technology and retirement (e.g. Buse 2009). As for item 3, the focus in HCI is on family-based interactions and how it feeds into the individual's motivations and use of technology. While many studies that put the family at the core of the interaction exist, it is hard to find studies that connect a family's practice of technology to the 'wider historical, cultural and social phenomena', much less one that has a focus on ageing adults.

Items 4, 5 and 6, with their language of choice points, trajectories and the concept of 'developmental risk' have not been the concern of HCI and ageing thus far. It may be that their relevance has not been demonstrated. Thus, this chapter aims to uncover how making these concerns salient can result in rich new areas of understanding in research on older adults and their technology use. It can also help in shedding light on some difficult areas of research with older adults such as systematically addressing heterogeneity. To aid in the discussion, a quadrant analysis will be conducted and the implications of each quadrant dissected for its potential value for research on older adults and mobile technology.

The Gerotech Clock

Diagram 1 maps age and wellness against the intended purpose of mobile technologies. The Y-axis is the age continuum, from younger to older users. The X-axis is a wellness continuum, with perfect health to the left and death on the right. 'Wellness' is chosen as an axis, as opposed to just 'health', for two reasons: firstly, the concept of 'wellness' encompasses social, mental and physical well-being; secondly, it references a common language with geriatrics when assessing the health of older adults. Overall, 'wellness' is of key importance when discussing the capacity of older adults to operate computing devices.

The Y-axis intercept is set at 65 years old. This is somewhat arbitrary, as age has been shown to be a poor predictor of life status or health status. However, the chosen intercept is in accordance with the World Health Organization's (WHO) convention for the definition of 'ageing' persons (World Health Organization 2000). Furthermore, it is the official age of mandatory retirement in Singapore and thus carries some weight as a marker of change in social contexts.

Taken together, these axes connect the lifespan and health. Against this background, we can examine the course of a person's relationship to technology as mediated by these factors. The four quadrants of analysis are:

I. Unwell-young users
II. Well-young users
III. Well-old users
IV. Unwell-old users

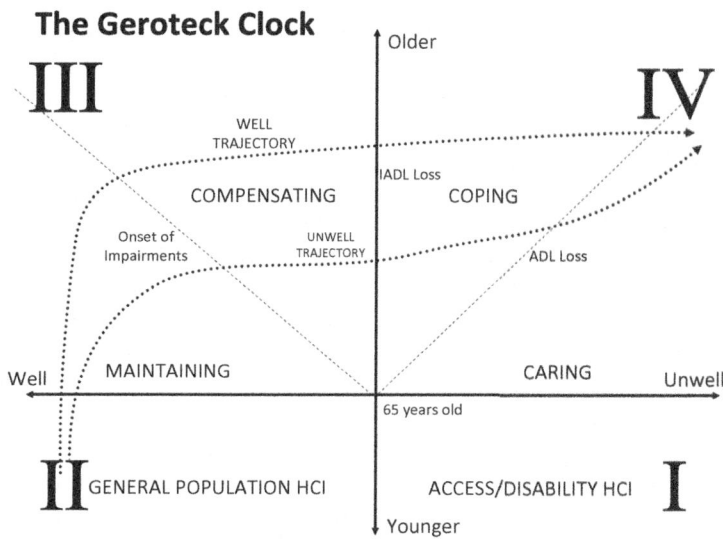

Diagram 1 Quadrant analysis of users by wellness and age

Each age-wellness combination results in markedly differing user requirements. Most of HCI research is focused on and tested with the well-young users in Quadrant II. This quadrant encompasses research with children, youth and adults who are statistically within the normal range. The unwell-young quadrant, Quadrant I, is the area of HCI concerned with disability or accessibility HCI. In this quadrant, the goal of technology is to augment or enable physical and cognitive functioning, such as with augmented speech devices or specially designed keyboards for low-vision users.

I have named this diagram the *Gerotech clock* because an individual's life trajectory passes through the various quadrants clockwise in a somewhat predictable order. A healthy life begins in Quadrant II, spends some time in Quadrant III and ends somewhere along the rightmost periphery of Quadrant IV, depending on the age of death.

Researchers of ageing and technology have observed that older adults are far from being a homogenous group that can be conveniently lumped into simple age and gender groupings (see Burdick and Kwon 2004; Charness and Boot 2009). Looking at the Gerotech clock, it is clear why this is so – at any age point, an older adult can potentially be in one of four very different health statuses. Furthermore, individuals will take different paths through their lifespan. Successful, healthy agers (on the *Well Trajectory* line) will spend the majority of their life in the leftmost quadrants, with a compressed period of morbidity before death. People who suffer a stroke will suddenly find themselves in Quadrant IV (on the *Unwell Trajectory* line) and spend their remaining years coping with a late onset of disability. Sometimes the transition occurs gradually, as with debilitating conditions such as osteoarthritis that can begin when a person is in his/her 40s.

Thus, the life course perspective offers an opportunity to capture the extreme heterogeneity of the 'ageing process', in the verb form, as opposed to examining 'older adults' as a homogenous, undifferentiated whole. While this is a benefit, it also requires adjustments in research methodology. Qualitatively, this necessitates the careful study of transitions between life statuses, the understanding of choice decision-making points and, finally, the resulting changes in life trajectories. Quantitatively, tools for analysing user trajectories over time are needed in HCI. Typically, cross-sectional, age-grouped studies are used to understand age-related changes. The main drawback of this study design is that it cannot account for individual differences. In this space, more longitudinal, within-subject studies are called for. In gerontology, Dykstra et al. (2005) used multilevel modelling, a statistical method that permits the simultaneous study of group and individual effects, to study changes in loneliness over time.

To the best of my knowledge, no studies exist in HCI that examine the relationship between older adults and technology in a similar manner, either qualitatively or quantitatively. Arguably, studies crafted with this approach in mind have the potential to produce rich findings, as has been the case in geriatrics and gerontology. This is further discussed below in section 'Compensating'.

The emphasis on trajectories does not preclude the structuring of the ageing process into four distinct but interdependent and consecutive phases. The next section expands on these four areas and explores the extent to which they have been addressed in current HCI research.

Maintaining

Quadrant III represents well-older users. However, there is significant heterogeneity in the age of onset and type of age-related impairments experienced by older adults. This argues for a further division of Quadrant III into two subgroups, to recognise that while some older adults have to cope with age-related impairments, there are also those who continue being cognitively and physically unimpaired well into their 80s. This distinction highlights the so-called successful agers (Rowe and Kahn 1997). These are older adults who experience little or no age-related impairment, or even if they do, they report no negative fallout as a result. The definition of 'successful agers' is still under debate, but Ng et al. (2009) offered one definition that balanced both biophysical and psychosocial criteria. Their definition comprised five criteria for successful ageing: good/excellent self-reported mental health status, independence in activities of daily living (ADL), minimal depressive symptoms, engagement in at least one social activity and one productive activity and finally a high level of life satisfaction. This study found that 28.6 % of elderly Chinese adults in Singapore fulfilled all of these criteria and fit the definition of successful ageing.

Therefore, technologies targeted at well-older users should not be focused on issues of impairment but, rather, be orientated towards the 'maintenance' of successful ageing. After all, these are older adults for whom no or minimal age-related adaptations are needed, and they merely require support for other transitions in life that are associated with advanced years. Examples here include grandparenting support (Vutborg et al 2010; Hutchinson et al 2003) or understanding the changes in social and information and communication technology (ICT) landscape that are associated with retirement (Buse 2009).

Due to the absence of 'troubles' for this category of older adults, they rarely receive explicit attention from HCI researchers. However, as will be discussed shortly, there may be cause to study this group, particularly as they pertain to later developments in the life course.

Compensating

For obvious reasons, the existence of the 'Maintaining' category does not mean that researchers can ignore the onset of impairments. As much as successful agers exist, so too do older adults who experience vision impairment, reduced auditory sensitivity or other such common markers of advancing age. However, these are not pathological conditions and can be quite effectively compensated for with access technologies such as hearing aids and vision correction tools.

In general, compensation methods have been extensively studied in mobile technology for older adults – cognitive compensation via reduced complexity or touch compensation via increased size of interface forms. The bulk of older adult technology accessibility guidelines address this space. However, these are responses to older adults as a static group. If we include the life course perspective in studying compensation methods, we would have to look further back at the successful agers and ask how onset of impairments has changed the way they use technology.

The age differences in smartphone adoption rates offer a departure point to begin investigations. In Singapore in 2012, only 15 % of residents aged 60 and above were using smartphones. Among the younger 50–59 year olds, smartphone ownership was at 46 % (InfoComm Development Authority of Singapore 2012). Further research is needed to understand this large gap. Do cohort effects alone explain the difference, or is there a more complex interaction between age-related impairment, cohort effects, coping mechanisms and personal history causing these differences? As mobile phones form a key method for the delivery of wellness interventions, the retention of mobile phone usage would be highly desirable.

As mentioned earlier, the life course perspective would call for the search for transitions and choice points – the crucial junctures at which undesirable consequences can be avoided. In the case of lung disease, this is the concept of 'developmental risk' points. In HCI, it seems that the idea of 'developmental favour' might be more productive to expanding our understanding of the relationship between ageing users' continued use and adoption of technology and the features of the technology itself. For example, we already have evidence that previous work experience with computers is a stronger predictor of technology acceptance than age (Wilkowska and Ziefle 2009). Building on that understanding, we might also ask how experience with computer programming changes users' ability to cope with error recovery, something older adults are often find difficult. Perhaps certain impairments are more strongly predictive of the lack of mobile phone adoption.

There is some hint in the literature that this will be a productive research direction. In a review of touchscreen interaction techniques for older adults, Motti, Vigoroux and Gorce recommend that researchers always document users' previous experiences with technologies and the internet, as well as the types of age-related impairments that each user is experiencing at the time of sampling (2013, p. 132). Otherwise, the heterogeneity of older adults' background and health conditions lead to highly variable, non-generalisable results. In short, a comprehensive technology history for older adult users might be the HCI equivalent of the health history used in epidemiology.

Overall, the potential impact of these studies would lie in learning how better to preserve or encourage technology use among older adults.

Coping

In Quadrant IV, we see the transition from well older adults to unwell older adults. While this transition can be operationalised in many ways, a concrete measure of this transition is the loss of personal independence via disabling conditions. The field of geriatrics provides two useful measures of disability – the inability to perform instrumental activities of daily living (IADL), followed by the inability to perform ADL. The former category includes a wide range of self-care activities, such as shopping, paying bills and driving. The second category consists of six specific items – bathing, grooming, changing, feeding, functional mobility and toilet hygiene. Both categories indicate the need for caregiver help, but the loss of ADLs is clearly the more serious loss.

In the Singapore Burden of Disease 2009 study, the top three conditions associated with disability in those aged 65 and above are ischaemic heart disease, stroke and diabetes mellitus, with Alzheimer's disease and other dementias rising in importance (Phua et al. 2009). These diseases often lead to the loss of mobility and cognitive impairments that signal the loss of the ability to perform IADLs and ADLs.

Thus, the deployment of mobile technology in this category must cater to a moderate to high level of disability that may have started in some form in the 'Compensating' phase, but has now progressed beyond full recourse. Thus, 'Coping' and technologies that aid coping come to the fore in this quadrant.

In this target space, research into gerotechnology includes things such as cognitive orthotics (Pollack 2002), speech augmentation tools or robotics for at-home mobility (Kidd and Breazeal 2008). We also see the onset of telemonitoring in all its forms – from medical personnel administered home care to remote elder monitoring linked to non-resident family caregivers (Winters 2002). The loss of IADLs also triggers the need for home care automation.

It is in Quadrant IV that caregivers emerge as a critical user group. Hitherto, helpers of older adults were mentioned in research studies as part of the 'Maintenance' and 'Compensating' landscape, but were never given prominence. However, as IADLs are lost to ageing adults, it is the caregivers who step in to take over these functions. In Singapore, these are most often adult children and their spouses (77 %), followed by spouses of the care recipient (15 %) (Malhotra et al. 2012). From legal to organisational matters, the loss of IADLs is a handy signal that a caregiver is shouldering day-to-day responsibilities. Hence, the potential mobile technology needs in 'Coping' are much more than the issues of access that we saw in 'Compensating'. There are also legal, financial and organisational issues. This need is echoed in a study on digital inheritance in the family. Massimi and Baecker (2010) found that legal and ethical ownership issues complicate inheritance of digital artefacts and concluded with this statement: 'When designing domestic technologies, we must remember that these home technologies will always have at least two users: the primary user, and the inheritor' (p. 1829). When seen as an example of domestic technology in the caregiving context, the mobile phone of the future should also have two users, with all the attendant affordances. This idea is already starting to filter into commercial practice. In 2015, Facebook implemented options permitting users to elect a digital executor who is authorised to change or delete the profile of a user once proof of death has been received (Cooper 2015).

Cognisance of this principle would open up the need to study mobile technology from a greater societal perspective. Hence, the study of caregivers and 'Coping' is potentially a place where the family and its use of technology become a lens through which we can understand older adults' use of technology, both as individuals and as part of the larger legal and ethical framework they operate in.

Caring

The needs of the caregiver come to the fore in the final section of Quadrant IV. As in Quadrant III, the more extreme ends of the age and wellness continua also result in a qualitatively different user group. As the six key ADL abilities are lost, users in this extreme section are now older adults who are moderately to severely disabled and require a full-time caregiver. Cognitive and physical impairments of older adults increase the likelihood that the caregivers are now the main operators of every technology except the most effortless devices. Hence, this section is named 'Caring', for the technologies that support caregiving and for the caregivers who operate them. Impaired older adults are not often a target design group, possibly because the cognitive or physical impairments are too challenging. Researchers creating artefacts for this target user group often adapt by allocating complex device operations to 'secondary' stakeholders, i.e. the caregivers.

But are these truly the secondary users? For example, Cohene et al. (2005) designed an interface for dementia patients to view family memories. The content of the interface, videos and stills of family images were solicited from family members. The evaluation of the interface included the family members being present. If the artefact were to be productised, it is clear that the role of the 'secondary' user will in fact be to supply content. In fact, Cohene et al. observed from this case study that there was 'significant impact' on the family arising from their participation in the interface design process. They conclude that 'in this project, user-centered design does not just entail focusing on an end user. It involves…how to provide support to *all individuals* affected by a pervasive disease' (p. 1303, emphasis mine). The call goes beyond additional affordances for family members – it requires technology interventions to account also for the emotional and support needs of the caregiver. This case study was probably the first to indicate that the concept of 'secondary' users or stakeholders in the context of design for impaired older adults may be in need of further examination.

A later point of challenge arose in the role of caregivers as people who offer technological support. Gerling et al. (2011)) designed and implemented an 'exergame' for frail elderly in a nursing home. The game was conceptualised, as most digital games tend to be – for stand-alone and potentially unaccompanied gaming sessions. This is sensible in a nursing home environment, as the diversionary value of games lies in their ability to beneficially occupy residents without the involvement of overstretched caregivers. Still, it is hard to conceive of digital products that do not involve maintenance and set-up. Gerling et al. note this limitation in their conclusions: "The gaming situation of older adults in nursing homes should be considered…ad-hoc play without extensive set up routines should be explored" (p. 62:7). If a digital game is meant to provide diversion therapy, but requires set-up and support from caregivers during gameplay, are the goals of the design met even when an older adult is being entertained? It seems there is a need for language to define and support the balancing of multiple needs in this relationship.

Finally, a challenge to the idea that caregivers are 'secondary' users is that sometimes they are actually the *key operators* of certain types of mobile technologies that are meant to support eldercare. In this regard, we see most often bedside telecare systems or online health information or mobile applications that are inaccessible to bedridden elderly but are primarily used by caregivers. In such situations, it is difficult to differentiate who is the main beneficiary of technology. Caregivers benefit by improving their caregiving options, while older adults in turn benefit from improved quality of care. This begs the question, are the beneficiaries of a technology automatically synonymous with the users? I posit that, particularly in the caregiver-care recipient relationship, the answer is 'no' and that the careful study of caregiving contexts will help to enrich mobile technology researchers' ideas about who the users actually are.

Are there more 'Caring' needs of caregivers and older adults that are not currently being met? Some other underserved care needs include practical concerns for older adults such as end-of-life decision-making and creating legal documents such as wills. Preparing for end-of-life using technology is as much a concern for the caregivers as it is for the older adult (Foong 2008). For the caregiver, the same set of legal and financial transition tools that were mentioned earlier in 'Coping' may be useful. When the notion of continuity between the phases of the Gerotech clock is superimposed with the life course perspective, it can be clearly discerned that transitions over time should be a prime concern for mobile technology design and has been neglected thus far.

Other practical needs include just-in-time information resources for at-home nursing care or drug management systems for patients who have polypharmacy concerns. More holistic needs may include respite care systems and emotional support systems for caregivers. Older adults, even while bedridden, can still engage in therapeutic, creative activities, as long as their reduced abilities have been catered for (Kübler-Ross 2011). As seen in the dementia case study mentioned earlier, mobile, haptic-linked technologies are well suited to the supply of supported, small but repetitive activities that characterise therapy for older adults with impairments.

Implications of the Life Course Perspective for the Design of Mobile Technologies

In summary, the life course perspective calls on HCI researchers to think of the entire lifespan of older adults, rather than of discrete groups and conditions. There is clear evidence that cohort effects can change the requirements of mobile technology, but the preceding analysis has highlighted some other ways that the life course perspective can be augmented to further influence research in HCI.

Specifically, the Gerotech clock offers a handle on the diverse heterogeneity of abilities that characterises the older adult population. By dividing the population according to age *and* wellness, four basic phases of older adults and their relevant technology needs were examined. At the two ends of the older adult wellness spectrum, it was shown earlier that there is a need to study the transitions from full health to impairment and then from independence to dependence, with a view to designing technologies that support these transitions. Complemented by the Gerotech clock perspective, the life course approach proposes the study of human agency and developmental risk/favour as the goals of research on technology and the elderly. Crucially, it informs HCI research on older adults by pointing to the interdependence of lives within the caregiving nexus of the family. The discussion on family caregiving for older adults revealed points where current HCI conceptions of the user, and the primacy of users, need further work. With this consideration in mind, I will now discuss some issues that are salient in the Singapore situation and the implications for mobile technology design.

Dementia and Its Effect on the Burden of Home-Based Caregiving

The impact of dementia is holistic and pervasive. Dementia has been characterised as the archetypical geriatric condition – if a person has dementia, she/he is likely to experience some combination of all other geriatric conditions. Since the numbers of dementia patients among the elderly are rising worldwide, dementia is a useful lens by which to examine how age-related pathologies affect the life course and by extension family caregivers.

Worldwide, by 2020 there will be 50 million people diagnosed with dementia (Brodaty et al. 2011). All dementias are incurable, although progress can be slowed down with drugs. The onset is hard to detect, although it usually becomes clear that there is a functional defect after about 2 years of struggling with increasing difficulties with short-term memory. Other symptoms of dementia may include behavioural difficulties such as wandering, sundowning and aggressive episodes. As the disease progresses, people with dementia will require more care for increasing hours of the day. Depression also tends to co-occur in demented patients. People with dementia (PWD) live from 3 to 12 years after diagnosis (Kua et al. 2014).

Clearly, home-based, informal caregivers of PWD have a massive burden on all fronts – economic, psychological and social (Schulz and Martire 2004). In Singapore, the average cost of caregiving for dementia patients can easily outstrip the income of the caregiving household (Chong et al 2013). In a study among family caregivers (Seng et al 2010), 27.2 % of caregivers expressed feelings of burden. In this study, the top three scores for caregiver burden on the Zarit Burden Interview were for 'feeling stressed between caring for your relative and trying to meet other responsibilities for family or work', feeling 'your relative is dependent on you' and feeling 'that you should be doing more for your relative' (ibid, p. 760). In what may be peculiar to predominantly Chinese Singapore, which places a premium on filial piety, worries about caregiving performance emerged as a key factor in caregiver burden (Lim et al 2014). As well, a multinational systematic review of dementia caregivers observed that 'female caregivers bear a particularly heavy burden across cultures, particularly in Asian societies' (Torti et al. 2004). Singapore data reflects a similar female bias among informal caregivers, with 60 % being female (Malhotra et al. 2012).

By 2050, Singapore's projected population will have 35 % of people aged 60 and above. At the same time, it is projected that this is the year where the parental support ratio will go from the current 10:1 to just 2:1. The parental support ratio is the number of people aged 18–64 versus the number of people aged 65 and above (Singapore Department of Statistics 2014). Thus, the emerging picture is of a female-biased group of caregivers who are overburdened on all fronts, caring for disabled elderly over a long period of time. In about 40 years, these are the caregivers who would have grown up with mobile technologies and will be likely to be more open and able to utilise these technologies for their needs.

Unmet Needs in Elderly Caregiving

In a qualitative, focus group-based study among family caregivers, Vaingankar et al. (2013) summarised caregivers' perceived unmet needs as the following: information, financial support, accessible and appropriate services and emotional and social support. The type of information needed was both of the 'basic' variety and of the 'timely' variety. Participants of the study also needed information on the many types of healthcare support services available. While complex, these are all needs that mobile technology, in combination with good content, can provide. Information services exist, but they are 'out there' in the internet and require time and effort to transform into timely knowledge.

It is also not clear if such systems have met caregiver needs. In a meta review of 'tech-based' information systems for caregivers, (Thompson et al. 2007) found that while three out of four studies reported statistical significance post-intervention, the overall effect on caregiver depression, although positive, was non-significant. A larger systematic review of networked technologies supporting caregivers of people with dementia (Powell et al. 2008) characterised the outcomes as 'moderate' and inconsistent across 15 papers. Clearly, more work needs to be done to connect caregivers and the information they need in timely and useful ways.

Foreign Domestic Workers as Caregivers

Thus far, the discussion has centred purely on family caregivers. However in Singapore, 49 % of informal caregivers are assisted by foreign domestic workers (FDWs). Of these workers, 79 % were hired expressly for the purpose of helping with care of the elderly. The hiring of a FDW often stands between care at home and institutionalised care (Tew et al. 2010).

However, the utilisation of FDWs often represents a problem with communication barriers and inadequate eldercare skills. Beyond these practical difficulties lie some complex interactions between the presence of the FDW and family caregivers' own role in the caregiving relationship (Østbye et al. 2013). The full extent of the ambivalence around the presence of a migrant worker in the Singapore home is discussed in detail elsewhere (see Yeoh and Huang 2009). The situation is best summarised as one that is potentially explosive, with its mix of uneven power relations, communication difficulties and caregiver stress. Cases of caregiver abuse and worker abuse are but symptoms of this largely hidden tension. As the population ages and more older users require caregivers, it is imperative that the study of mobile technology for caregivers must at the very least account for FDWs as part of the caregiving system.

A search of key HCI research databases, the ACM Digital Portal and IEEE Explore, reveals that no studies include FDWs as part of the caregiving ecology. As previously mentioned, most studies focus on the older adult as the 'main' user and refer to 'family' and 'caregivers' as the other parties the system of care surrounding older adults. However, such an approach does not reflect the grim realities on the ground.

Research Agenda

In light of the preceding discussion on caregiving, we can identify three strategic nodes in the research agenda for mobile technologies for the elderly:

A. An understanding of how technology needs develop as the older adult transitions from independence to dependence. The life course perspective should inform this and pay special attention to the identification of developmental risk/favour, transitions and life trajectories.
B. Research into caregivers' specific needs, and how these needs conflict or co-exist with the needs of older adults, thereby developing methods for designers to explicate and resolve conflicting user needs in the caregiver-care recipient relationship.
C. A taxonomy of caregiving relationships and technology uses that can help researchers identify and meet needs.

Item A looks at the life course of both the older adult and the care recipient, and attempts to trace how needs develop as independence are lost. In so doing, it has the potential to begin technological support at a time when care recipients can supply more input into the affordances they want preserved. Taken together, B and C aim to provide a language to describe the many possible dimensions of caregiving and how each role may have different requirements. Finally, item C also speaks to the greater HCI community in terms of developing explicit ways to address the concept of user and stakeholder and to cater to diverse needs within the same application.

Conclusion

To propose the inclusion of a new approach into an existing field of research requires some speculation regarding its benefits. The life course approach is not without its drawbacks, the most difficult of which is the problem of separating age, period and cohort effects. Nevertheless, this chapter has brought together demographic and epidemiological data to help illuminate a previously unexplored area in the development of mobile technologies for older adults. The data has highlighted points of urgent need, and the life course approach, operationalised through the Gerotech clock, has pointed out the initial steps to be taken to tackle the resulting research questions.

As with all adoptions of methodologies into HCI, there will be points of debate as to the appropriateness of application of a method that arose in gerontology, to a field that originally focused on the efficacy of computing systems. I believe I have highlighted a mere subset of issues at the intersection of these fields. The substance of these debates will emerge when more researchers apply the life course perspective to gerotechnology.

I would like to end with a welcome to those debates, because they would signal that more researchers are taking on this approach. Ultimately, it would mean that more researchers are employed in meeting the urgent challenges of an ageing population.

Acknowledgement For their feedback on early versions of the Gerotech clock: Dr. Lydia Seong and Alice Chin of the Agency for Integrated Care, A/P Sun Sun Lim, Prof. Shengdong Zhao and my colleagues at the NUS HCI Lab and, finally, attendees at the Mobile HCI 2014 Workshop on Interfaces for Older Adults, where the Gerotech clock was first presented.

References

Ballard, B. (2007). *Designing the mobile user experience*. Chichester/Hoboken: John Wiley & Sons.

Ben-Shlomo, Y., & Kuh, D. (2002). A life course approach to chronic disease epidemiology: Conceptual models, empirical challenges and interdisciplinary perspectives. *International Journal of Epidemiology, 31*(2), 285–293.

Benyon, D., Turner, P., & Turner, S. (2005). *Designing interactive systems: People, activities, contexts, and technologies*. Essex: Pearson Education.

Brodaty, H., Breteler, M., DeKosky, S. T., Dorenlot, P., Fratiglioni, L., Hock, C., & De Strooper, B. (2011). The world of dementia beyond 2020. *Journal of the American Geriatrics Society, 59*(5), 923–927.

Burdick, D. C., & Kwon, S. (2004). *Gerotechnology: Research and practice in technology and aging: a textbook and reference for multiple disciplines*. New York: Springer Publishing Company.

Buse, C. E. (2009). When you retire, does everything become leisure? Information and communication technology use and the work/leisure boundary in retirement. *New Media & Society, 11*(7), 1143–1161.

Charness, N., & Boot, W. R. (2009). Aging and information technology use potential and barriers. *Current Directions in Psychological Science, 18*(5), 253–258.

Chong, M. S., Tan, W. S., Chan, M., Lim, W. S., Ali, N., Ang, Y. Y., & Chua, K. C. (2013). Cost of informal care for community-dwelling mild–moderate dementia patients in a developed Southeast Asian country. *International Psychogeriatrics, 25*(09), 1475–1483.

Cohene, T., Baecker, R., & Marziali, E. (2005). Designing interactive life story multimedia for a family affected by Alzheimer's disease: A case study. In *CHI'05 extended abstracts on Human factors in computing systems* (pp. 1300–1303). New York: ACM.

Cooper, D. (2015). Facebook lets you choose what happens to your profile after you die. http://www.engadget.com/2015/02/12/facebook-digital-executor-service/. Accessed 17 Feb 2015.

Dykstra, P. A., Tilburg, T. G. van, & Gierveld, J. de J. (2005). Changes in older adult loneliness results from a seven-year longitudinal study. *Research on Aging, 27*(6), 725–747.

Foong, P. S. (2008). Designing technology for sensitive contexts: supporting End-of-life decision making. *Proceedings of the 20th Australasian conference on computer-human interaction: designing for habitus and habitat* (pp. 172–179). New York: ACM.

Gerling, K. M., Schulte, F. P, and Masuch, M. (2011). Designing and evaluating digital games for frail elderly persons. *Proceedings of the 8th international conference on advances in computer entertainment technology* (pp. 62:1–62:8). ACE'11. New York: ACM.

Hutchinson, H., Mackay, W., Westerlund, B., Bederson, B. B., Druin, A., Plaisant, C., & Eiderbäck, B. (2003). Technology probes: inspiring design for and with families. *Proceedings of the SIGCHI conference on Human factors in computing systems* (pp. 17–24). New York: ACM.

Hutchison, E. D. (2010). *Dimensions of human behavior: The changing life course*. Thousand Oaks: Sage.

InfoComm Development Authority of Singapore. (2012). Annual survey on InfoComm usage in households and by individuals for 2012. http://www.ida.gov.sg/~/media/Files/Infocomm%20Landscape/Facts%20and%20Figures/SurveyReport/2012/2012HHmgt.pdf. Accessed 6 Nov 2014.

Kidd, C. D., & Breazeal, C. (2008). Robots at home: Understanding long-term human-robot interaction. *Intelligent Robots and Systems, 2008. IROS 2008. IEEE/RSJ International Conference on* (pp. 3230–3235). Piscataway: IEEE.

Kua, E. H., Ho, E., Tan, H. H., Tsoi, C., Thng, C., & Mahendran, R. (2014). The natural history of dementia. *Psychogeriatrics, 14*(3), 196–201.

Kübler-Ross, E. (2011). *To live until we say good bye*. New York: Simon and Schuster.

Lim, W. S., Cheah, W. K., Ali, N., Han, H. C., Anthony, P. V., Chan, M., & Chong, M. S. (2014). Worry about performance: a unique dimension of caregiver burden. *International Psychogeriatrics/IPA, 26*(4), 677–686.

Malhotra, C., Malhotra, R., Østbye, T., Matchar, D., & Chan, A. (2012). Depressive symptoms among informal caregivers of older adults: Insights from the Singapore survey on informal caregiving. *International Psychogeriatrics, 24*(Special Issue 08), 1335–1346.

Massimi, M., & Baecker, R. M. (2010). A death in the family: Opportunities for designing technologies for the bereaved. *Proceedings of the SIGCHI Conference on Human Factors in Computing Systems* (pp. 1821–1830). New York: ACM.

Motti, L. G., Vigouroux, N., & Gorce, P. (2013). Interaction techniques for older adults using touchscreen devices: A literature review. *Proceedings of the 25 ième conférence francophone on l'Interaction Homme-Machine* (p. 125). New York: ACM.

Ng, T. P., Broekman, B. F. P., Niti, M., Gwee, X., & Kua, E. H. (2009). Determinants of successful aging using a multidimensional definition among Chinese elderly in Singapore. *The American Journal of Geriatric Psychiatry, 17*(5), 407–416.

Østbye, T., Malhotra, R., Malhotra, C., Arambepola, C., & Chan, A. (2013). Does support from foreign domestic workers decrease the negative impact of informal caregiving? Results from Singapore survey on informal caregiving. *The Journals of Gerontology Series B: Psychological Sciences and Social Sciences, 68*(4), 609–621.

Pacey, A. (1983). *The culture of technology*. Cambridge: MIT Press.

Phua, H. P., Chua, A. V., Ma, S., Heng, D., & Chew, S. K. (2009). Singapore's burden of disease and injury 2004. *Singapore Medical Journal, 50*(5), 468–478.

Pollack, M. (2002). Planning technology for intelligent cognitive orthotics. In *Proceedings of the sixth international conference on artificial intelligence planning and scheduling* (pp. 322–332). Toulouse: The AAAI Press.

Powell, J., Chiu, T., & Eysenbach, G. (2008). A systematic review of networked technologies supporting carers of people with dementia. *Journal of Telemedicine and Telecare, 14*(3), 154–156.

Rowe, J. W., & Kahn, R. L. (1997). Successful aging. *The Gerontologist, 37*(4), 433–440.

Schulz, R., & Martire, L. M. (2004). Family caregiving of persons with dementia: Prevalence, health effects, and support strategies. *The American Journal of Geriatric Psychiatry: Official Journal of the American Association for Geriatric Psychiatry, 12*(3), 240–249.

Seng, B. K., Luo, N., Ng, W. Y., Lim, J., Chionh, H. L., Goh, J., & Yap, P. (2010). Validity and reliability of the Zarit burden interview in assessing caregiving burden. *Annals of the Academy of Medicine, Singapore, 39*(10), 758–763.

Singapore Department of Statistics. (2014). Population trends 2014. http://www.singstat.gov.sg/Publications/publications_and_papers/population_and_population_structure/population_trend.html. Accessed 14 Nov 2014.

Stoller, E. P., & Gibson, R. C. (Eds.). (2000). *Worlds of difference: Inequality in the aging experience*. Thousand Oaks: Pine Forge Press.

Tew, C. W., Tan, L. F., Luo, N., Ng, W. Y., & Yap, P. (2010). Why family caregivers choose to institutionalize a loved one with dementia: A Singapore perspective. *Dementia and Geriatric Cognitive Disorders, 30*(6), 509–516.

Thompson, C. A., Spilsbury, K., Hall, J., Birks, Y., Barnes, C., & Adamson, J. (2007). Systematic review of information and support interventions for caregivers of people with dementia. *BMC Geriatrics, 7*(1), 18. doi: http://doi.org/10.1186/1471-2318-7-18.

Torti Jr, F. M., Gwyther, L. P., Reed, S. D., Friedman, J. Y., & Schulman, K. A. (2004). A multinational review of recent trends and reports in dementia caregiver burden. *Alzheimer Disease & Associated Disorders, 18*(2), 99–109.

United Nations. (2002). World population ageing. http://www.un.org/esa/population/publications/worldageing19502050/. Accessed 4 Nov 2014.

Vaingankar, J. A., Subramaniam, M., Picco, L., Eng, G. K., Shafie, S., Sambasivam, R., & Chong, S. A. (2013). Perceived unmet needs of informal caregivers of people with dementia in Singapore. *International Psychogeriatrics, 25*(10), 1605–1619.

Vutborg, R., Kjeldskov, J., Pedell, S., & Vetere, F. (2010). Family storytelling for grandparents and grandchildren living apart. *Proceedings of the 6th Nordic conference on human-computer interaction: Extending boundaries* (pp. 531–540). New York: ACM.

Wilkowska, W., & Ziefle, M. (2009). Which factors form older adults acceptance of mobile information and communication technologies? In A. Holzinger, & K. Miesenberger (Eds.), *Human computer interaction for eInclusion* (pp. 81–101). Berlin/Heidelberg: Springer.

Winters, J. M. (2002). Telerehabilitation research: Emerging opportunities. *Annual Review of Biomedical Engineering, 4*(1), 287–320. Retrieved from http://www.annualreviews.org/doi/abs/10.1146/annurev.bioeng.4.112801.121923

World Health Organization. (2000). The implications for training of embracing: A life course approach to health. http://www.who.int/ageing/publications/training/en/. Accessed 6 Nov 2014.

Yeoh, B. S., & Huang, S. (2009). Foreign domestic workers and home-based care for elders in Singapore. *Journal of Aging & Social Policy, 22*(1), 69–88.

Index

A
Access, 2, 5–7, 17, 21, 23–29, 51, 52, 55, 57–59, 64, 80, 82, 84, 85, 87–89, 98, 110, 113, 114, 132–134, 138, 142, 144, 152, 154, 155, 162, 171, 173
  to technologies, 5, 52, 85, 89, 142
Active mediation, 38, 44, 131–133, 142
Activities of daily living (ADL), 171, 173, 174
Adolescents, 2, 130, 133, 156. *See also* Youths
Adverse activity displacement effect, 42
Affective bonds, 6, 75
Affordances, 96, 133, 142, 173, 174, 178
  for family members, 174
Age, 15, 17, 19, 21, 22, 55, 77, 78, 89, 97, 99, 100, 102, 113, 131, 133, 134, 139, 140, 142, 143, 147–148, 152, 166–172, 174, 176, 179
Ageing
  nations, 167
  phenomena, 168
Ambient technologies, 166
Approach, 3, 4, 14–16, 20, 29, 41, 66, 75, 95, 96, 124, 131, 133, 134, 142, 166–168, 170, 176, 178, 179
Augmented speech device, 170

B
Biographies, 166, 167

C
Cambodia, 75–80, 84, 85, 87, 88
Caregivers, 138, 152, 158, 159, 162, 173–178
Carry principle, 166

Child development, 16
Children, 53, 131–134, 137–140, 144
  school-aged, 16, 27, 29, 130
Chinese
  education system, 16
  society, 14–17, 19, 28, 29
Choice points, 168, 172
Cognitive, 131, 139, 142, 166, 167, 172–174
Collective experience of family members, 149
Communication
  devices, 134, 142
  interpersonal, 52, 53, 95, 158
  practices, 76, 79, 94, 105–106, 114
Connected presence, 100, 102
Connectivity, 80, 85, 93, 101, 105, 116, 119, 122, 166
Consumerism, 18
Contact
  direct and unmediated, 82 (*see also* Direct and unmediated contact)
  long distance, 82, 148 (*see also* Long-distance contact)
Content
  pornographic, 35
  risk, 41
Context aware, 167
Cost, 5, 6, 16, 20, 30, 53, 57–59, 64, 75, 79–81, 83, 86, 102, 114, 117, 151, 154, 176
  of technology, 10, 34, 43, 46
Courtship, 44
Co-using, 131–133
Co-viewing, 38, 131–132
Cultural, 95
  probes, 4, 55, 56

D

Death, 167, 169, 170, 173
Dementia, 176–177
Demographic, 144
Design, 7, 8, 56, 66, 103, 165–179
Developed countries, 165, 166
Development of interpersonal skills, 53
Diaspora, 147–148, 162
Digital
　artefacts, 173, 174
　citizenship, 131
Direct and unmediated contact, 82
Disabilities, 167
Domestic
　helpers, 5, 51–67
　responsibilites, 37
　technology, 173
Domesticating household ICTs, 37
Dying, 167

E

Education, 5–7, 13–30, 35, 36, 38, 40, 42, 43, 45, 46, 77, 80, 83, 84, 88, 94, 97, 110, 117, 120, 131, 135, 137, 142–144, 156, 157, 160, 179
Elderly, 166, 167, 171, 174–178
Emerging technologies, 95–97, 101. *See also* Technologies, emerging
Entertainment, 18, 117, 144
Epidemiological, 179
Ethnography, 4, 16, 19, 76, 167
Experience, 2, 5–7, 17, 19, 20, 22, 38, 39, 41, 45, 46, 52, 54–62, 64–66, 74, 77, 78, 80, 95, 98, 112, 113, 115–119, 124, 132, 137, 147–162, 166–168, 171, 172, 176

F

Facebook, 6, 34, 58, 66, 67, 79, 84, 85, 99, 100, 103, 111, 112, 114–121, 123, 124, 173
Familial obligation, 75, 86, 112. *See also* Obligation, familial
Family(ies)
　identity, 52, 54
　interaction, 2, 93, 95, 101, 103
　members working conditions, 96
　multi-local, 84, 85
　norms, 103
　nuclear, 85, 131
　story, 54, 62, 65
　storytelling, 5, 51–63, 67, 105

Family–based interactions, 168
Feature phones, 17, 130
Filipino mothers, 7, 147–163
Foreign domestic worker as caregivers, 177
Framework, 3, 4, 15, 18, 21, 29, 41, 75, 95, 106, 112, 168, 174
Frequency of transnational family communication, 96

G

Gendered parenting norms, 161
Geriatric care, 166
Geriatrics, 166, 169, 170
Gerontology, 166, 170, 179
Gerotech clock, 7, 169–171, 175, 176, 179
Global interconnection, 148
Globalization, 94
Grandparenting, 168, 171

H

Haptic extensions, 166
Health
　challenge, 168
　issues, 129
　measures, 168
Healthcare, 82, 167, 177
Healthy and safe media habits, 130
Human computer interaction (HCI), 166–168, 170–172, 175, 176, 178, 179

I

IADL. *See* Instrumental activities of daily living (IADL)
Impact of mobile phones on education, 21
Impairments, 167, 171–175
Indian migrants, 76, 77, 88
Indonesia, 34, 35, 52, 130, 135
Indonesian Muslim mothers, 5, 33–47
Infocomm Development Authority of Singapore, 172
Information and communication technologies (ICTs), 52
Instant messaging, 27, 95, 101
Instrumental activities of daily living (IADL), 173
Interaction, 2, 4–6, 19, 55, 65, 74, 93, 95, 98, 101–103, 109–124, 129, 131, 132, 137, 138, 163, 168, 172, 178
　face-to-face, 98, 101
Interface design process, 174
International students, 97, 103, 110, 115

Index

Internet
  cafes, 79
  e-learning applications, 35
  filtering software, 35
  literacy program, 35
Internet-based phone calls, 79
Interpersonal communication, 52, 53, 95, 158
Intimacy, 76, 82, 88, 89, 104, 149
Islamic values, 35, 37, 44, 45

J
Jakarta, 130, 134

K
KakaoTalk, 95, 99, 100, 102–105

L
Learning, 14–16, 21, 22, 26, 28, 35, 110, 137, 140, 159, 172
Left-behind family members, 84, 86, 96, 121, 162
Life
  course, 74, 167, 168, 171, 176, 178
  satisfaction, 54, 171
  statuses, 170
  trajectory, 168, 170
Long-distance contact, 82
Longitudinal, 133, 170
Low-wage migrant workers, 105

M
Marriage, 85
Media
  beliefs and perceptions, 35
  content, 4, 34, 35, 36, 38, 45, 47
  diaries, 113, 114, 124
  habits, 130, 138, 143
  industry, 34
  landscape, 96
Mediated parenting, 102, 148, 149, 151, 157, 161, 162
Mediation
  active, 38, 44, 131–133, 142
  restrictive, 131–133, 140, 142
Medicine, 168
Methodology, 19–20, 77–78, 97–98, 113
Migrant
  mothers, 150, 161
  students, 110 (*see also* International students)
  workers, 111
Migration theory, 74
Mobile, 25–26, 28, 76, 78–80, 82, 83, 88, 102–105, 129, 133–137, 143, 148, 150, 152–161, 175–179
  applications, 134, 175
  communication, 1–8, 14–16, 18–20, 27, 29, 53, 82, 98, 103, 110–112, 122, 129–144, 148, 152–159, 162
  computers, 165
  dependence on, 151, 154
  desire for, 29
  and education, 18, 21
  and internet technologies, 89
  parenting experiences, 162
  phone pentration and ownership, 17, 20, 25, 26, 78–80, 88, 152
  phones, 1, 5, 13–30, 35, 52, 53, 57–60, 64, 66, 67, 75, 78–84, 87, 88, 94, 99, 102, 111, 114, 115, 118, 120, 123, 148, 151–155, 160, 166, 172, 173
  subscriptions, 26
  technologies, 15, 16, 30, 76, 81, 89, 93, 95, 106, 166, 169, 175, 177–179
  telephony, 75, 80, 87, 94
Mobility and cognitive impairments, 173
Moral economy, 106, 112, 121, 124
Mothers, 37
Motivations for use of mobile technology, 167
Muhammadiyah, 36, 39, 40
Multi-local families, 84, 89

N
Needs in elderly caregiving, 177
Negative effects of mobile phones on education, 21, 24
Networked technologies, 177
New-borns, 168
Non-formal and formal systems of learning, 16

O
Obligation, 15, 37, 43, 45, 75, 81, 124
  familial, 75, 86, 112
Old age, 15, 166
Older adult, 175

Online
- risks, 130–132, 137
- health information, 175
- games, 132

Orkut, 79, 84

P

Paradoxes, 150–161

Parental, 138–140
- mediation of children's internet use, 34, 133
- obligations, 15, 37, 43, 45, 75, 81, 86, 112, 124

Parenting
- mediated, 53, 102, 148–162
- remote, 7, 152, 157, 161

Parents
- rural, 5, 28
- suburban, 5

Personal computers, 99, 152

Philippines, 52, 76, 86, 151, 160, 162

Physical
- cognitive functioning, 170
- distance, 28, 102

Pornographic content, 34, 35, 44, 133

Portable computers, 166

Practice, 2, 4–6, 14, 16, 18, 20, 28, 35, 38, 39, 41, 76, 79, 83, 84, 87, 94, 95, 98, 101, 106, 112, 130, 132–134, 138, 141, 143, 149, 161–163166, 168, 173

Precollege study abroad, 94, 105

Primary user, 173

Privacy in communication, 154

Professional, 78, 80, 85, 88

Public health policies, 168

Q

QQ instant messenger, 25

Quadrant analysis, 169

R

Religious
- beliefs, 34, 38, 39, 41, 47
- ideals, 39

Remittances, 75–76, 81, 86–89, 104, 106

Remote parenting, 152, 157, 161

Risky online behaviors, 133

Romantic relationships, 28, 29

Rural parents, 5, 28

S

School-aged children, 16, 27, 29, 130

Sensor enabled devices, 166

Sex, 35, 138, 139, 142, 160.
  See also Intimacy

Shared communal space, 44

Sharing experiences, 52, 54, 57, 58

Singapore, 52, 110–114, 116–124, 151, 153–155, 159, 162, 163, 166, 169, 171–173, 176–178

Single male rural migrants, 75

Situational, 158, 167

Skills in using technology, 88

Skype, 79, 80, 84, 85, 99, 100, 102, 104, 114, 115, 117, 118, 120, 123

Smartphones, 166

Social
- capital, 76, 87, 123
- characteristics of these, 29
- media platform, 27
- mental and physical well-being, 169
- networking, 22, 79, 84
- relationships, 29, 75, 76
- support, 52, 53, 177

Socioculturally oriented, 96

South Korea, 94, 132

South–South migration, 75, 77

Spatial and temporal conditions, 148–150, 153, 155, 157, 158, 162

Strategies, 25, 28, 29, 77, 84, 86, 94, 106, 131–133, 138–140, 143, 150, 154
- behavioural, 166

Study machines, 14

Successful agers, 171, 172

Suharto, 34, 36

Surveillance, 18, 89, 102, 116, 122

Symptoms of dementia, 176

T

Tablets, 7, 14, 57, 58, 114, 129, 134–140, 142, 144, 166

Targeting choice behaviours, 168

Technological affordances, 96

Technologies, 14, 15, 18–20, 29, 74–76, 80, 83, 84, 86–88, 93, 98, 100, 110–112, 122–124, 129, 148, 149, 151–155, 159, 162, 166, 171–177
- access to, 52, 85
- ambient, 166
- emerging, 95–97, 101, 130
- interventions, 172, 174
- networked, 177

Technology domestication theory, 2–8, 18, 96, 111–112
Theory
    migration, 74
    technology domestication, 2–8, 18, 96, 111–112
Tools for analysing user trajectories over time, 170
Touchscreen interaction techniques, 172
Transnational, 74–76, 93, 98–102
    capital, 86
    families, 81, 84, 93, 94, 96–103, 105, 106, 111, 112, 124, 148, 149, 151, 153
    mobility, 93, 94, 148

U
United States (US), 38, 94, 110, 111, 129
University, 20, 30
Upward mobility, 5, 42

Urbanized, developed countries, 166
User
    group, 166, 167, 173, 174
    requirements, 170
User-centered computing systems, 167

V
Vietnam, 1, 110, 113, 114, 116, 117, 119–123

W
WeChat, 25, 27, 67
Weibo, 27
Wellness, 169, 172, 174, 176
World Health Organization's (WHO), 169

Y
Yahoo messenger, 79, 80, 85–86
Yogyakarta, 39
Youths, 14, 17, 98, 170

The manufacturer's authorised representative in the EU is Springer Nature Customer Service Centre GmbH, Europaplatz 3, 69115 Heidelberg, Germany. If you have any concerns regarding our products, please contact ProductSafety@springernature.com

Printed and bound by CPI Group (UK) Ltd, Croydon, CR0 4YY

25/03/2026

02078174-0003